FIGHTING SPIRIT

THE AUTOBIOGRAPHY OF FERNANDO RICKSEN

FERNANDO RICKSEN

WITH VINCENT DE VRIES

TRANSLATED BY MICHIEL BLIJBOOM

This edition first published in 2019 by
ARENA SPORT
An imprint of Birlinn Limited
West Newington House
10 Newington Road
Edinburgh
EH9 1QS

First published in Great Britain in 2014

www.arenasportbooks.co.uk

ISBN: 978-1-909715-90-5
eBook ISBN: 978-0-85790-812-4

First published in the Netherlands in 2013 by Voetbal International B.V. as
Vechtlust: Het Bizarre Leven van International Fernando Ricksen

British Library Cataloguing-in-Publication Data
A catalogue record for this book is available on request from the
British Library.

Designed and typeset by Polaris Publishing, Edinburgh

Printed and bound by CPI Group (UK) Ltd, Croydon, CR0 4YY

CONTENTS

To Veronika – and everyone else who believed in me

And to Isabella

ACKNOWLEDGEMENTS

Fernando,

 People say you were a nutcase.

 People say you were completely out of your mind.

 People say you were a troublemaker, an unguided missile.

 People say you couldn't deal with other people.

 But after all our talks at your cosy home in Maaseik, I knew better. You were a lambkin, just as your former team mate Barry Ferguson always says. A fighter, never running away from his responsibility. A fighter who was willing to face even the biggest challenge, even one of the most cruel diseases in the world: MND.

 Thanks for being so open and honest. You will always be an example to others.

 At your funeral in Glasgow, after six years of battling MND, Veronika, your lovely wife, said: here in Scotland they already knew that you were a star, long before you left us. Well, you are still a star, but now one that we can see every night, high up in the sky.

 She is so right. Keep shining, Fernando. We will never forget you.

I would also like to thank the following, in alphabetical order. You have all been a huge help in making this book what it is.
Pamela Aalbers, Michiel Blijboom, Peter Burns, Marieke Derksen, Linde Dreessen, Barry Ferguson, Esther Goergen, Bjorn Goorden, Andy Goram, Michiel Holsheimer, Gordon Irvine, Eddy van der Ley, Michael Mols, Victor Morgan, Carol Patton, Laetitia Powell, Anneke Ricksen, Pedro Ricksen, Bobby Singh, Goffe Struiksma, Eric Verhoeven and Veronika Veselova.

Vincent de Vries

FOREWORD

I'M NOT A MORNING person. Anyone who knows me, or who has had to put up with me over the years, will testify to that.

So it's fair to say Fernando Ricksen was my worst nightmare.

I'd be sitting there, at Murray Park, having a cup of tea and some breakfast, just minding my own business, taking it easy. The way I like it. And then the doors would burst open and in he'd come. Always at 100mph. Fernando did everything at 100mph – it's just the way he was.

Anyway, I'd roll my eyes and think to myself, 'Oh shit, here he comes – bang goes my peace!'

The truth is he didn't shut up. Ever. The guy was completely hyperactive and always had to be getting up to something or other. He couldn't sit still.

So, yes, I admit it, there was a sinking feeling in the pit of my stomach every time I saw him bolt in through those doors with that big grin on his face, like a kid on a sugar rush. He was a total pain in the arse; but, deep down, I loved the guy for it.

So I can't begin to explain the sense of shock I felt when I received the first message about his TV appearance in Holland, during which he revealed he was unwell. My first reaction was to dismiss it; there must have been some kind of mistake. But as the texts kept coming, I realised it must be true. My old teammate had contracted motor neurone disease.

Now don't get me wrong, I knew right away it didn't sound good. But it was only when I went away and researched it online that I realised the full extent of what Fernando was lat ahead for him. A disease they couldn't cure? It was just too horrible for words.

No one deserves to suffer in that way. But Fernando of all people? Sometimes this world is too cruel, because you will never meet a more kind-hearted guy. He was a crazy guy, but one with a heart of gold. There was never a dull day with the Dutchman.

People made him out to be a lunatic because of all the stuff he got up to, but he wasn't anything of the sort. I remember him as a big kid who didn't have an off button – and that's hardly unusual in this line of business. Paul Gascoigne was the same type of character and there have been plenty of others. But that didn't make him a bad guy and certainly not the kind of monster he was sometimes made out to be.

He was a beast, for sure – especially on the pitch – a hungry animal that needed to be fed on silverware. That's why it was so good to have him in the team. Fernando may not be the world's best footballer, but he was a born winner. A fighter. That's why he was always so popular among Rangers fans. They love a guy who throws himself into the cause with utter commitment, doing everything he could to win. He loved the club and the club loved him.

In his final months, I think he knew that. The whole football world was behind him.

Honestly, you could not meet a nicer guy than Fernando. And I don't say this because he said I was the best footballer he ever played with – which, looking at all of his former teammates, is an enormous honour for me.

It always made me laugh when I heard some of the nasty stuff people would say about him. These were the thoughts of absolute idiots who didn't know the first thing about him as a human being. Yes, Fernando's image suffered because he was capable of doing some stupid things on and off the pitch. But aren't we all? And, mind you, I am quite envious of some of those 'stupid things'. I mean . . . waking up next to Jordan, are you kidding me? That's the stuff legends are made of. And Fernando, truly, is a legend.

He was a fiery guy on the park too and sometimes he got carried away there as well. But he wasn't out there trying to hurt or maim people; he was just one of those guys who got so wound up in a game that sometimes the heat of the moment got the better of him.

But that same enormous drive led to international honours with Holland, silverware for Rangers and Zenit Saint Petersburg and his induction into the Rangers Hall of Fame. Some people have said that his induction is because of his illness, but that's as callous as it is untrue. The man won prizes for the club and he was our captain. If you have done that, you belong in the Hall of Fame.

The way he lived his life, the way he played on the pitch, was always on the edge. He was whole-hearted in everything he did and I love the guy for that.

By the time I came back to the club from Blackburn for my second spell at Ibrox, Fernando was the team captain and I saw a huge change in him as a player. He thrived on the extra responsibility and from moving into midfield from full-back. I thought we complemented each other really well and I enjoyed playing beside him. We thought we could take on anyone together.

Still, I didn't realise just how bad his diagnosis was until I read up on it. It took me a full week until I found the strength to have a look at the TV footage of him, talking for the first time about MND. That's because not everybody is as brave as Fernando. Anyway, after reading all those text messages and having done my research, I found myself doing a strange thing. I put my iPad down and went into the next room to lie down with the kids and watch TV. Something inside me made me need to be close to my family.

The proudest part of being a father is watching your kids grow up and playing a part in their development into adults. That's what being a parent is all about. But Fernando only had a few years with his daughter. And that's the saddest thing of all.

I guess it just proves a point: you've got to live life to the full because you don't know what's around the corner. And at least that's what Fernando has done. He has lived his life to the full. You find all the proof you need of that statement in this book.

And I will remember him the way he was. With that big smile. About to ruin another bloody breakfast.

Barry Ferguson

ONE

LITTLE CHICAGO

'SO, TELL ME, WHAT is it exactly that you have achieved in your life?'

Now that was a question I hadn't seen coming. I almost choked on my glass of water when the psychologist at the Sporting Chance Clinic asked me this, and not because it was water.

Didn't this man read newspapers? Didn't this man watch TV? Didn't this man follow football?

Okay, a few days ago I had been on the rampage – again. This time, on a flight to Johannesburg. I couldn't deny it. But, hey, I was Fernando Ricksen, highly successful professional football player. Twelve caps for the Netherlands. Loaded. Capable of bedding any woman I wanted. Winner of seven – did you get that, shrink? – *seven* major trophies with Glasgow Rangers. Voted Best Player of the Scottish Premier League – by my colleagues. Best Player, meaning just as much a hero as Paul Gascoigne, Mark Hateley, Brian Laudrup, Ally McCoist and Henrik Larsson.

How about *that*?

And this man was asking me what I had achieved?

I was the captain of Glasgow Rangers, one of the best and biggest football teams in the whole of Britain. Only the real big shots in football will ever have the privilege of wearing the captain's band in a team like Rangers. Big shots like, well, me.

This guy is nuts, I told myself. Asking me what I had achieved, the sheer idiocy of the question. No respect whatsoever. It was a joke!

At that very moment I knew it: this whole Tony Adams clinic wasn't for me. What the heck was I doing here? Had I really come to the place voluntarily? I remembered having had doubts beforehand. I'd been right!

But, being the confident person I thought I was, I explained to him that loads of people were envious of me. Okay, minor detail: Paul Le Guen, Rangers' new manager, had just kicked me out of the squad for 'indecent behaviour', which in this case meant running through an aeroplane on a flight to a training camp in South Africa – stark naked and pissed as a parrot.

Nevertheless, stadiums full of people would love to swap places with me. In their eyes I had a career to die for. They, in other words, simply admired me for all I had achieved.

And I wasn't exaggerating.

'Oh?' the psych said, leaning backwards and folding his hands behind his neck. He had a completely different opinion. My self-image sucked. Big time.

I offered him a question mark.

'Yes,' he said. The word sounded as if it came straight out of a ventilator. Then the volume knob was turned to the left. He started whispering. 'Listen. Your club doesn't want you any more. Your wife wants to leave you. Basically your life has gone down the drain. Completely.'

Those words had an enormous impact on me. I listened in silence. Because, deep down, I knew he was right. Of course he was right. As a football player I had made it – no doubt about it. Even a blind man could see that. But as a human being? Not quite.

I had to face it: I had been drunk and disorderly for years now. I had kicked my way through life like a football hooligan with an insatiable thirst. Thanks to that, my life was in tatters. It was just as the guy with the pencil who was sitting in front of me said. I knew it, but I'd never wanted to show it to anyone. Scared shitless to lose all the respect I had gained over the years.

2

I know it sounds odd, but I was glad that on that sunny morning in Hampshire in July 2006 the doctor came to this verdict. More important: I was happy that he shared it with me. I felt relief, more than anything else. Finally someone had the guts to stick a needle into the balloon. Or, in this case, a sharp pencil. I felt liberated. Free. As if a huge weight was falling off my shoulders. This really was what I needed.

I decided to stay. Motivated at last. As I said earlier, I had come to the clinic voluntarily, but at the time I didn't think much of it, to tell the truth. The clinic's big boss Peter Kay had advised me to seek help here, but I genuinely thought I didn't need any. I believed I was doing all right. Well, that's what it's like when you live in your own fantasy world. How wrong I was . . . I *did* need help, and I needed it fast.

So, as I was sitting there, regarding the natural beauty of Forest Mere, Liphook, I realised that this could be *the* chance to leave Never Never Land, with all its destructive seductions, for good and start facing reality. There was no time to lose, otherwise I would lose more than time alone, meaning my beloved Graciela and my just as beloved Rangers.

There and then I took the decision that would change my life. I was ready to fight myself. 'Deal,' I said to the psych, while stretching out my arm. He shook my hand.

Here, on this beautiful estate, I would be reborn. Just as Kay hoped, when he advised me to check in to the clinic.

'For the next few weeks I'm gonna do exactly what you tell me,' I said to the doctor.

He smiled, and nodded. 'Good to hear that, son.' He told me I wouldn't regret my decision. To start with, I wasn't the first addicted sports hero here. There had been truckloads of them before me. And each of them had walked out of the clinic as a better person. Cured, sane.

I could follow in their footsteps, the psychologist said. And he was right, or so it seemed. After a few difficulties in the beginning, I was more than happy to leave the clinic as a reborn man. A lot less egotistical than when I had arrived only four weeks earlier.

Little did we know . . .

I mean, the feeling I had was one of total euphoria. It just wouldn't last. I didn't know there were more terrible things lined up for me, over the horizon, and things would get worse. Much worse.

*

It must have puzzled a few that, of all people, I ended up in rehab, battling booze and reshaping my mental self. Several eyebrows must have been raised in Hoensbroek, the quiet town in the Dutch province of Limburg where I was born on 27 July 1976, with the name of Fernando Jacob Hubertina Henrika Ricksen (I was named after the hit single by Swedish pop group ABBA, who happened to be my mother's favourite band). Everyone in and around Eikstraat, or Oak Street as you would say in English, knew me as a quiet and even polite child.

In nursery I never caused any trouble. I was shy and well behaved. Every time the headmaster of Saint Paulus – Limburg is a predominantly Catholic region, hence my four Christian names – called my mother to tell her one of her kids had been a bit of a naughty boy, she knew who he meant straight away.

It was always Pedro, my younger brother. Never Fernando. And, indeed, Pedro was a bit of a mean bastard. Always pushing his luck, always trying to get away with things, always looking for trouble. Totally unlike me.

I was a good boy. And that didn't change when I went to primary school. Every single year I ended up with good results. Strange to say it now, but I think I was a perfect child.

Pedro, who is only three years younger than me, was completely different. A whirlwind. Always on the rampage. If my mother wanted to visit friends or relatives and mentioned that she would be bringing Pedro with her, the visit would be cancelled. Nobody wanted Pedro in their house. Quite understandably, I have to confess.

Pedro loved the negative effect he had on people. He thought it was cool to be the bad boy. And boy, was he bad! Even towards me.

4

I remember playing with my brand new Commodore 64, which I'd received from Santa. My friends and I were gathered around the computer and the television screen having heaps of fun, until Pedro pulled the plug. Just because he felt like it.

I don't know if you remember the Commodore 64, but you needed tapes to upload the games. Needless to say Pedro cut those on more than one occasion, the sneaky bastard.

He didn't give a toss whether my stuff was brand new or not. In those days, a Game Boy was the coolest thing a boy could have. It allowed you to play games wherever you were. And I was so damn proud of mine! Still, it didn't take Pedro long to destroy it. I still remember where it happened: in the car, on our way to the Piccolo camping site in Domaso near Lake Como, our annual holiday spot. He simply broke it – and with that he broke my heart too. God, without my beloved Game Boy, the drive to Italy took an eternity.

As if driving to the campsite wasn't boring enough, being the experienced truck driver he was, Dad never felt the need to stop along the way. We just drove straight to Italy, without any nice and cosy intermissions. Fourteen hours in an old Ford Taunus (which was like the Ford Cortina in the UK) without air con, it felt like a barbecue in hell – but without any sausages. Between Limburg and Italy we had one, maybe two, brief stops, but that was it. Daddy Huub, who was in fact my stepfather but we always called him Dad, wanted to reach the campsite as fast as possible. Not least because the whole family was waiting there already. Personally, I never got it. I mean, we stayed there for six bloody weeks, so what was the rush?

At times, I had to beg to stop for a pee.

'Not yet,' Dad always said.

By the time my bladder was ready to explode, he would give in and pull over. But not, like normal people do, in a parking area. He'd just stop on the hard shoulder! There, with all the motorway traffic speeding past, I had to go. And I had to go fast, Dad said. With the pee still dripping from my willy I had to jump in the car again, as the driver said we had no time to lose.

No time to lose! The old Ford was so heavily loaded that we

barely made it on to the motorway again. It was so chock-a-block with luggage and people, the pressure on its wheels must have been enormous.

Oh, and apart from us humans, there was a dog on board as well. We didn't want to put Max, our beloved Cocker spaniel, into a kennel, so he went with us to Italy. I had this drooling animal sitting next to me for the full fourteen hours, which drove me nuts. That, and the caravan dragging behind us, meant we could hardly pick up any speed, so the trip seemed to take for ever.

The only distraction I had was my Game Boy. For as long as it lasted, that was. Why the hell did Pedro have to destroy it? And why couldn't he sit still for one bloody minute?

I cried a lot on those occasions, but Pedro didn't feel guilty at all. If anything, he looked as if he was enjoying the situation. He always picked on me, always.

'Nando!' he yelled one day. 'Turn on the radio! I made a request for a record, especially for you!'

I was excited. It was nice he'd done that for me. Full of anticipation I sat in front of the radio, listening to a local station from Heerlen, a city not far away.

And then it came: 'And here's a song especially for Fernando Ricksen from Hoensbroek.' I was thrilled. Until I heard it.

The song was 'Huilen Is Voor Jou Te Laat' by Corry en de Rekels. Or, in English: 'Crying Comes Too Late For You' by Corry and the Rascals. The Corry in question was a blonde hairdresser from the province of Brabant, and it was the kind of shit music grandmothers like. A Dutch attempt to make a Tammy Wynette-style country ballad, but much, much worse. Check it out on YouTube . . . The fact that it spent a total of 41 weeks in the Top 40 says a lot about the Dutch and their taste, I guess.

Anyway, it was a crap song and it made me cry. Appropriate title, after all!

Pedro used to end up in fights, all the time and everywhere. He had arguments at school, on the street, and, yeah, even at our local football club EHC.

He'd always been a lot crazier than me. That's why my parents chose him to be Prince Carnaval: a nutter dressed as a jester who jumps out of a box at the opening evening of the local carnaval club.

I need to explain something here. Carnaval, four days in which people dress up, drink gallons of beer and dance the conga for hours, is a huge deal in Limburg. The ideal stage for a bullshit artist like my brother Pedro. Being Prince Carnaval would make him the centre of attention. Perfect! It was just that he was too young. So my parents had to come up with a substitute.

Me.

I didn't like it at all. I was too shy, too introverted for that wacky stuff. But I didn't want to let my parents down. Besides: what did I have to lose? Nothing.

So, before I could say 'confetti', I was dressed up in a white uniform with matching gloves and, er, tights. On top of my head I had the traditional red and white bicorn hat with a long pheasant feather. To complete the picture I had a silver sceptre in my hand and some well-earned medals around my neck. Well, any prince would have been allowed to walk around with those decorations, as they were just handed over by one carnaval club to the other.

So, as much as I hated it, I jumped out of the box. Just as I was told. I even managed to smile, believe it or not. Well, if you really want to, you can check it out yourself, as it was captured on camera. My mother was so proud she immediately hung the photo of her Boy Prince on the wall. And for years and years I had to walk past the damn thing.

Much later I asked Pedro why he'd always been so unfriendly to me. Why he did all those things that made me feel uncomfortable, that made me cry. 'I was envious of you,' he confessed. 'You were everybody's favourite little boy. I hated that.'

Nowadays Pedro is one of my best and closest friends. And I have to say that it has had some benefits, being the brother of this little brat. For instance, I never had to be scared of anyone, because as much as he was unpleasant to me he also defended me on more than one occasion. Anyone stupid enough to lay a finger on me could expect a good hiding from my little hooligan brother.

From the moment I went to Saint Jans College, a high school on Patersweg (Priest Road) in Hoensbroek, things changed. Because I did. Training with the professionals of Fortuna Sittard, all grown men, on an almost daily basis, did something to my body. It made me a different guy. Stronger – both physically and mentally.

And all of a sudden things were different. Now it was Pedro who would ask me to help him to solve the odd problem. The poor little chap really thought he could beat up some of my classmates, who were all three years older than him. So what do you do as a big brother who has gained a muscle or two at the Fortuna gym? You beat up the bastards who are bullying your kid brother. Despite the fact that it had been him who had started stirring the shit most of the time.

Where the Ricksen family was living at that time, fisticuffs were part of daily life. It was the end of the eighties and we had moved to Heerlerheide, a notorious area in the northern part of Heerlen, a grim city close to the German border. They didn't call Heerlerheide 'Little Chicago' for nothing. I mean, you couldn't get a bus in our neighbourhood, because the drivers were too scared to enter the area!

Before then, the local bus company did have a few stops in Little Chicago. But after being hit by flying bricks and concrete missiles every single day, all of a sudden they decided not to take the risk any more.

Pedro and my parents still live there, and, from what I understand, it's still a tough neighbourhood. Unemployment and criminality galore. Angelique, Pedro's wife, never goes out for a walk at night. Too dangerous.

The sound of sirens is the soundtrack of my years in Little Chicago. It was completely normal to see a police car or an ambulance racing through the streets. So I didn't really think much of it one afternoon when I was sitting on the couch, just home after a holiday in Spain with Pedro, and heard the sirens. It gave me a buzz. It was top amusement. And, hey, guess what? This particular time we had front row tickets!

But, er, why were the cops lining up in front of *our* house? And what was the meaning of the red and white ribbons at either end of the street? I asked Pedro, but he didn't have a clue either. Point is: we were both just back from our holiday and no avid readers of the local newspaper. So whatever was going on in our neighbourhood, we didn't know about it. The only thing I did know was that all of this was not because of a stolen apple.

Maybe it was murder! Maybe someone had been killed! Quite possible, in Little Chicago, with its German junkies.

But, no, it wasn't about that. They were looking for a kid – a kid with a gun. Eyewitnesses had seen him, earlier that day, at a roundabout. The boy had been threatening a fellow driver. It seemed serious, hence the calls to the cops.

Turned out I knew that kid.

It was Pedro.

Enter the blue brigade, storming into our humble abode like the barbarian hordes of Attila the Hun. My father, bless him, tried to stop the invasion with the assistance of Max who, you may remember, was a Cocker spaniel. As they tried to shoot him – the dog, not my father – the old man backed off. He didn't want to be responsible for a dead Cocker spaniel.

Yelling and cursing, they put their handcuffs on poor Pedro's wrists. Ladies and gentlemen, we've got him! And off they went again – didn't even ask for a coffee.

It turned out they had the right man too. Yes, it had been Pedro that afternoon at the roundabout, pulling a gun on another driver. A toy gun – okay, from a souvenir shop in Spain – but the thing looked surprisingly real. It was the type of pistol that John Wayne used to do the talking in most of his Westerns. Except this wasn't the Wild West, it was Heerlen. And Pedro wasn't exactly John Wayne.

Pedro wasn't Arnold Schwarzenegger either, so why he felt the need to whack a female copper at the police station, I don't know. As if the arrest itself wasn't bad enough. Anyway, my little brother ended up in jail that night. Dad had to get him out.

All in all he was left with a 250-guilders fine, which nowadays would be about £110. Oh, and they kept the gun.

The saga of Pedro's Pistol isn't the only weapons-related incident I have witnessed from a short distance. Let me introduce you to Maurice Rayer. We met in 1994, when he was playing with me at Fortuna. He was on loan from VVV, a club in Venlo. Beautiful guy – quite literally – who could score on and off the pitch, if you catch my drift. Needless to say I loved going out with this babe magnet.

Another ladies' man was Hans Kraay junior, of Brighton, er, fame. In his active years record-breaking red and yellow cards collector Kraay junior (his old man, Hans Kraay senior, was a famous Feyenoord footballer in the sixties) played for a string of clubs the length of the Great Wall of China, one of them being San Jose Earthquakes where he rubbed shoulders with a certain George Best. Anyway, good-looking blokes, those two. Perfect company for a night on the pull. Our tight little mob was completed by pint-sized Nigerian Tijjani Babangida, who would eventually end up at Ajax.

I can't remember which one of us was driving, but at a certain moment, in between pub visits, our car came to a sudden halt. No idea why. Neither did I understand why Hans all of a sudden left the car, yelling at the top of his voice. And why, for Christ's sake, was he carrying a . . . gun?

I knew he was mental. The whole of the Netherlands did. But this?

Hans went straight for a guy who was sitting on a bench. Completely out of control, fuming, like he was on the pitch.

It was like watching a B-movie in which the bad guy shouts, 'Your money or your life!'

And that was exactly what Hans screamed.

I, in the meantime, was almost wetting my pants. Not because I was scared, but because it was hilarious. Top comedy. It was a practical joke, of course. Everyone knew it was a joke. Everyone except the poor tramp, who had been sitting quietly on a bench minding his own business.

'Your money or your life.' To a homeless person. Geddit?

To make things worse, the bum actually *did* give his money to Hans. All three guilders of it. The poor bastard was scared shitless. And pretty short-sighted, it seemed, as the weapon Hans was waving at him was a water pistol from a pound store. A yellow one, on top of that.

Of course, Hans, being the gentleman he is, told the hobo he could keep the change.

My weapon of choice, at the time, was always a billiards cue. No, not to beat people up, but to play a game of libre! I was pretty good at it, I must say. Hopeless at snooker, but quite a champ when it came to this continental version of the game, with two white balls, a red one and a table without pockets. Once I even came third at the Dutch Championships. The fact that I won bronze was remarkable. You had to be at least eighteen years old to enter the competition. I wasn't. I was twelve.

It must have been great for the audience to see this little kid in his grand café outfit, hardly taller than the table itself. On more than one occasion I had to stand on my toes like a ballet dancer.

People would be in stitches when they saw me enter the arena, but within minutes there would be silence.

It must have been quite a sight, this little whirlwind going around the table, scoring one point after the other. I mean, I was smaller than the actual cue! In the end, nobody wanted to play against me any more. I was simply too good.

It was in the genes. My mother's father, Willem Szymiczek, was one of the best players in the country. He'd taught me every trick in the book. He was a fanatical coach, my grandfather. I remember analysing TV footage of important billiards tournaments with him, or going through one of his many books. Great memories.

Playing billiards was very rare for a boy of my age. At school I was the only one. But I didn't care. Every day after school I would run to my granddad's house because he had a billiards table there. Never played with other kids; always practised alone, or with him. Couldn't care about the other kids playing football in the street. My granddad's workshops, that was what counted!

As a young and talented billiards player, I managed to win piles of silverware. One day I was even rewarded with a week-long training session with the one and only Raymond Ceulemans. I took it for granted. Had never heard of the guy. My granddad literally had to explain that this Belgian bloke Ceulemans was the best billiards player in the entire world. 'He can teach you *everything*,' Granddad said, without even trying to hide his excitement. 'You'll learn more than I could ever teach you, Nando.'

Of course he was right, for Raymond Ceulemans was a legend. It's just that I wasn't really into worshipping sports heroes. The walls of my bedroom, for instance, were bare. No posters with pictures of football players, rock stars or hot chicks. Pedro's room, on the other hand, was covered in pictures of his favourite football club, Roda JC.

Every time the lot of us went to a Roda match, Pedro was determined to collect as many autographs as possible. Not me. I couldn't care less, thought it was childish.

'In a few years' time, people will ask me for my autograph,' I exclaimed, full of confidence.

What I did do, though, was wear replica football shirts. Always. But because we were not exactly rich, they happened to be poor quality ones. Fake-ish. Well, completely fake, to be honest. Official replica shirts were way too expensive for us. Hence the cheap Made in China rubbish I wore.

Apart from that, my mother knitted woollen football jumpers. She loved doing that. Between the two of us, Pedro and I must have had about seventy of the things. Personalised jumpers, too, with our own names – years before football clubs did stuff like that!

Apart from jumpers in the colours of Roda JC, Fortuna Sittard and Ajax, we had a lot of Italian ones: AC Milan, Inter, Juventus, AS Roma, Napoli . . . I wore them day and night. And if I didn't, it was because I was wearing my Dutch national team tracksuit. An official replica! I got it as a Christmas present and burst into tears when I first saw it. Albeit not as loud as when I fell on the pavement and ended up with a big hole in the trousers! I was inconsolable, until I realised that the knitting champion my mother was could fix it quite easily.

The fact that most of my jumpers depicted Italian clubs wasn't a coincidence. Due to our annual visits to Lake Como, I grew to love Italian football culture. I even started to buy that famous pink football paper, *La Gazzetta dello Sport*, despite my knowledge of the Italian language being limited to the words 'pizza' and 'pasta'. Staring at the pictures and all those beautiful names was exciting enough.

Every year, on one of the first days of our vacation, we used to go to Milan. To be precise: the famous San Siro stadium, which was like the Holy Grail to me. Its souvenir shop was the place where I parted with most of my 100-guilders holiday money. And most of the time on day two of the holiday! I didn't care, and neither did my mother. For her, the holiday couldn't begin until she had taken me to San Siro. Otherwise I would have been a nuisance – and she knew it.

'One day I'm going to play here!' I'd say, year in, year out, as I enjoyed the grandeur of the place so much. And of course I was joking there. Or was I?

Fast-forward fifteen years to 28 September 2005: Internazionale v. Glasgow Rangers, Champions League. I'd made it. I was playing in the stadium of my dreams. Dreams could sometimes come true! Although I have to say that in my fantasy the stadium was totally sold out. In reality it was empty, due to a UEFA punishment. And we lost, which was also not scripted by me. David Pizarro, Inter's Chilean wizard, came up with a 24-carat free-kick. The first time our goalie Ronald Waterreus saw the ball was on the TV footage afterwards.

The Ceulemans session wasn't a success. Three days into the week and I wanted to go home already. Not that I was homesick, oh no. I simply thought the whole thing was a waste of time. So I called my mother: 'You can pick me up now, Mum.'

Raymond Ceulemans was the Johan Cruyff of billiards. At least, that's what the world said – the whole world – but to me, the Johan Cruyff of billiards had another name. Granddad Szymiczek. A far better teacher than that Ceulemans chap, in my opinion.

Around my sixteenth birthday I had to make a choice between billiards and football. I'd become a pretty good footballer, and to get even better I needed to train on an almost daily basis. So that was it, as far as the noble game of billiards was concerned. My granddad didn't like the choice I made, but in order to become the best in one type of sport, I had to drop the other. Simple as that. Sorry, Granddad.

Thinking back, I sometimes wonder what would have happened if I had dropped football. No doubt I'd have been one of Holland's best billiards players. I mean, I already was! But, money-wise, have you ever heard of truckloads of hot girls swarming around a billiards player?

No, I made the right choice.

TWO

LAGER, LAGER

IT WASN'T THE MONEY that made me choose football: it was fun. And in those days clubs didn't pay *that* much for a youth player.

The pleasure started at the tender age of four, when I was trying to kick a ball on behalf of local football club EHC. Here, on the green and pleasant acres where 'Mr Fortuna' René Maessen started his career, people quickly noticed how talented I was. Not to boast too much, but I was so good I ended up in teams one age group above mine. On my players' card they simply changed '1976', my year of birth, to '1975'. Nobody would ask any questions. If opponents wondered why I was so much smaller than the rest of my teammates, we would tell them it was due to stunted growth. 'Poor little guy, just leave him alone. It's hard enough being so small.'

Once again, my talent was genetic. And as with billiards, it was all thanks to Granddad. He had been a football player himself – and a good one. In 1950, four years before professional football was introduced into the Netherlands, he even won the League when he played for Limburgia. They had faced Ajax in a play-off at the Olympic Stadium in Amsterdam and annihilated them 6–0. Granddad often told me what a fantastic afternoon it had been, with 60,000 spectators in the ground.

That became my dream. I wanted to be a champion too, just like him. I wanted to win trophies – be the best. The problem was,

15

I didn't just have that dream when I was in bed, I had it on the pitch too! My lack of concentration became notorious. Out of desperation, the coaches put me in the position where I could do the least damage. That's how I became a right-back.

I loved it, because it meant I was always close to my mother who attended every game and would warn me as soon as the ball was coming my way!

I was always focused on something else. Watching the birds – real ones, at that age – or fiddling with the label in my collar. I kept touching the bloody thing, over and over again. It almost drove my mother insane. She would yell at me: 'Nando, watch out! The ball's coming towards you!'

It took me no more than a split second to change from dreamer into hunter. And within the blink of an eye I had that same ball on my feet.

Well, after all I was a talent!

It turned into a pattern. Right after I'd kicked the ball away, the dreaming would start again. I would stop running and start playing with that damn label again. I didn't have a clue what was happening at the other end of the pitch. Not interested.

I wasn't alone though. Lots of my teammates were absent-minded a lot of the time. The big difference was that while they were still dreaming when they were in possession of that pumped-up piece of leather, I wasn't. As soon as I had the ball, I knew what to do. First thing being: not losing it to an opponent.

Not everyone appreciated it. I remember one little bloke walking towards my mum, in tears. I knew the guy. He was a friend of mine, despite the fact that he was playing for another club. That's why I didn't understand the tears. What had I done to him? I wouldn't kick him!

'Please, Mrs Ricksen . . .' he sobbed. 'Please ask Nando to let me go past him just once!'

I sympathised. Being a left-winger he was a pretty good dribbler, but I worked him out quite easily. Over and over again. So I blocked him every bloody time. After all, that was my job: to defend. He, on the other hand, wanted to enjoy the pleasure of running into the box and sending the ball towards the goal. At least once. Hence his plaintive request to my mother.

I didn't want any of it. Loved the guy, really, but he had to learn that defenders don't give presents to forwards. Ambitious defenders, that is. And I was ambitious. I wanted to become the best defender in, well, the world. So no sentimental drivel, please. I was working on my future here. If he wanted to go past me with that ball, he'd have to invent some good tricks. Like any good forward. Otherwise, try your luck at netball, mate.

In 1986, at the age of ten – or eleven, as it was known at EHC – I went to a Catholic club named RKONS. They were located in the southern town of Landgraaf, home of the annual Pinkpop festival. At RKONS, I was turned into a midfielder. That didn't do me any harm. On the contrary: it made me tougher, stronger, more confident.

The move from EHC to RKONS was because my parents had taken over a pub in Landgraaf. Yes, a pub! And I loved it.

The place became my living room. I mingled with the clientele, and sometimes even assisted as the place got crowded. Pedro and I collected empty glasses and rinsed them behind the bar. It was great fun. I went here, there and everywhere on a night like that – it was like being on the pitch.

Not a single empty glass escaped my notice. Later, I would swap them for full ones, of course, but not at that time. Not yet.

Ten years old, and already I was 'The Man' at the local pub. Walking around with an enormous stack of empty glasses, being noticed by everybody, I loved the attention, I can tell you.

Apart from the fun – and the added bonus of staying up late – it was profitable too. Every single evening we collected empty glasses we were rewarded with a handful of guilders, money that we used to spend the next day at the local toy shop. Pedro and I would buy cheap plastic shit, which was usually broken within hours.

Sadly, it lasted no longer than a year. Because my mother struggled to combine working in the pub with raising two little boys, my parents had to sell the place. And off we went, back to Little Chicago.

In the meantime, a small part of my dream had come true: I was playing for a professional football club. As a youngster, obviously, but still. I was a member of Roda JC's youth squad, and damn proud of it. For a boy from Limburg, more precisely this boy from Limburg, there were only two clubs that mattered: Roda JC and Fortuna Sittard. The other two professional ones, MVV and VVV, I couldn't care less about. So when, in 1988, a Roda scout approached my mother about me, I didn't have to think twice. Neither did she. The mighty PSV was interested too, but Mum didn't like the idea of me moving all the way to Eindhoven. I was too young, in her opinion. Well, bless her, I was happy with Roda too. It seemed to be the perfect first step on the ladder. All of a sudden I had to train four times a week instead of two, as was the case with RKONS, but that wasn't a big deal. If I wanted to make it, I would have to toughen up. Actually, I thought it was pretty cool: four training sessions a week.

As clubs weren't allowed to buy youth players from competitors, Fortuna Sittard didn't approach me any more, although I heard they were very interested in me. Tough luck, they simply had to wait . . . for a phone call from me, for instance.

And you won't be surprised to hear that the phone call came, right after the umpteenth argument with my coach Hans Fischer. I'd had enough and I wanted to go, the sooner the better. What a lousy coach he was! Couldn't teach me anything, with his ridiculously basic exercises. Hardly any of his youngsters have broken through on a national level. Enough said.

The thought of not being able to find a club any more never crossed my mind. Full of confidence I called Fred van Barneveld, youth coordinator at Fortuna Sittard, and explained the situation. I told him how much I wanted to play for Fortuna and how important it would be for my career. I wasn't making any progress at Roda, thanks to the crappy training. All they wanted me to do was 'kick and rush' – ideal for a football club in Britain maybe, but not for a

Dutch team, and especially not for a youngster in a Dutch team. I was eager to learn, so give me something worthwhile to learn!

Fred totally agreed.

Unlike at Kaalheide, Roda's stadium, there was a lot of focus on young players within the walls of Fortuna's ground, De Baandert. As was reported by Mark van Bommel – much later of PSV and Barcelona fame – who was my teammate in the regional youth squad, he kept asking me 'Why don't you come and play with us?' In fact, he posed the question so often I began to think he was taking me for a ride. So I stayed with Roda. In general I liked it there. And I was doing well, scoring about four goals per game! I was so good I was promoted to a higher age group again. So I felt like the King of Kerkrade. Well, not quite, but there certainly wasn't any lack of self-confidence!

All went well until about 1992. Around that time it occurred to me that the youth division was something of a necessary evil. They simply didn't care about us. For instance, we never got a chance in the main squad. Nol Hendriks, the wealthy owner of the club, preferred to buy new players rather than try out a few of his own youngsters. All he did was buy. And sell, of course; this banker loved to make a profit. At one point he even wanted to get rid of the entire youth department. Well, that about sums him up!

So, after one more of Mr Fischer's tricks – he didn't let me play with the older guys and at the same time refused to put me back into my own age group – I decided I'd had it with Roda. It was time to move on.

Fortuna were very happy when I called. Nevertheless, I had to play a few test matches. A formality. The games were part of a tournament somewhere in Limburg. And guess what? I won Player of the Tournament!

Now, I don't want to sound big-headed, but it didn't come as a surprise to me. Back then, I was already a member of the national youth team. With the famous orange shirt around my shoulders, I more than once ended up being one of the best players of the lot. No arrogance here, honest! Just facts.

I was sixteen when I signed my first contract with Fortuna. I earned 750 guilders with it and was over the moon. Two years later my youth contract was changed into a real one. I remember my mum and dad getting emotional when I told them the news.

I was a professional football player!

Despite my happiness, I kept my cool. There was a bigger goal to achieve, so I had to stay focused. Okay, it was wonderful to be able to earn money with my hobby, but I had to be aware of the fact that I'd just started to realise my dream. It was only the beginning. The hundreds of guilders I got were great, but it wasn't the Big Money I dreamed of. Yet.

Two other guys signed their first contract on the same day as me: Mark van Bommel and André van der Zander. The club put on a bit of a show, with the three of us signing a piece of paper on a table that was placed on the pitch. We felt like real professionals, proud of the beautiful yellow and green Fortuna shirt we were wearing. It was a magic moment.

'BELOFTEN BLIJVEN IN BAANDERT' was the alliterative headline in the newspaper. It meant that the club had contracted three of its most promising players.

My mother showed the clipping to everyone. She was so proud of me – and the fact that they'd finally managed to spell my name correctly. In the past, it had often been 'Riksen', or 'Hernando'. Not this time. At last, Fernando Ricksen had made the news!

To me, being signed by Fortuna was an enormous relief. It was great to have everyone in a major football club showing confidence in you . . . Well, everyone except head coach Chris Dekker.

He kept telling me that I was still a rookie, that it would be a long, long time before I'd really be of significance to the club, and that I may have to reach the age of 25 before I'd become a full-blown member of the first team.

I was flabbergasted. Was this the same man from the picture in the newspaper? The man who was standing behind me, grinning, while I was signing the contract? If he had any doubts, why did he give me a contract in the first place?

I didn't want any of this, so I told him, 'Tough luck if I have to wait that long. Tough luck – for you! You see, I work according to a schedule, my own schedule. It says: two more years at Fortuna and then my debut in the Dutch national team. Way before I turn 25!'

He laughed, thought I was joking.

But I wasn't. I was dead serious.

When I told him that, he laughed even louder. 'Forget about that, son,' he said, shaking his head. 'You'll never reach that far.'

When I noticed he wasn't joking either, I turned around and walked away, with my dad. It was useless talking to this man any longer. He simply didn't get it.

Didn't he know who he was dealing with? I was Fernando Ricksen, one of the biggest rising stars in the area. PSV wanted me, and so did Anderlecht. They recognised the fighter inside of me, the battler who would do almost anything to reach his goal.

'I'll get back to you when I'm 25!' Famous last words before I left Mr Dekker's office.

And, boy, did I prove him wrong! I was 24 when I made my debut in the Orange team, in an away game against Spain. I've never seen Dekker since then, which is a pity, as I'd loved to have seen his face!

I felt fantastic in my first days at Fortuna, hence my behaviour as a cocky show-off in Dekker's office. My many goals and assists were – what can I say? – mouth-watering. As a midfielder I scored about as many goals as a good centre-forward!

In all honesty it was all thanks to the amazing team I was in. Mark van Bommel, little Bart Meulenberg, Ronald Dassen, Ivo Pfennings, Freek de Winter and André van der Zander were top-class players and lots of them would end up in the first team. We were an amazing youth brigade, and together with our coaches John Walstock, Henk Duut and Cor Brom (a former head coach at Ajax) we lost just one game that season. Undisputed champions!

We were not just teammates, we were mates full stop. Friends, pals. Went to each other's birthdays. Downed our first pints of lager together. Glorious days, great memories.

Of the eighteen members of the squad, a mere sixteen went into town together on a Saturday night. No team building required – we were a team already!

Most of the time we went to the Peppermill, a big nightclub in Heerlen, right on the border with Germany. We had a ball there, drinking beer and staring at chicks from the side – we never set foot on the dance floor. In our opinion, dancing was uncool.

Mind you, we didn't have to chase the girls. As soon as they found out we were Fortuna players – and I confess we didn't exactly hide the fact – they were chasing us! But, with some of the other guys and myself already having girlfriends, we made a pact: whatever happens in the Peppermill stays in the Peppermill!

And that is exactly what happened. Nobody ever broke our deal, no matter how juicy the goings-on. So my beloved Desiree, who sent me one hand-written love letter after the other, never found out anything.

Mark, André and me were the first ones to make it into the main squad. We were just a bit better than the rest, especially André who could run like a racehorse. I always thought it was strange that, unlike Mark and me, he never really made it to the top. After three years of struggling at Fortuna, he went to Germany and ended up playing for clubs like Germania Teveren. What a waste.

And there are more examples of talented players who never achieved fame and fortune. Take, for instance, Rik Platvoet, whose surname funnily enough means 'Flatfoot'. He was centre-forward in various national youth teams and, my God, the boy could score! He was so good he kept Patrick Kluivert out of the team. That was until Kluivert, Ajax's greatest talent in decades, started to build some muscle. Only then could he take the place of Rik Platvoet, of whom we haven't heard much since. While Kluivert became a star at Ajax and Barcelona, Platvoet's CV includes names like Heracles, MVV, Emmen and VVV. Nice clubs for an average player, but Rik Platvoet was no average player.

Still, André and Rik are exceptions. Most of the time, somebody who has 'world class player' written all over him lives up to the expectations. Like, for instance, Clarence Seedorf. I couldn't believe my eyes when I had a shower with him after an under-16s match. Those legs! Concrete! And a six-pack to end all six-packs, un-be-liev-able!

He had the body of an adult, not that of a fifteen-year-old boy. Well, to be honest, he was an adult, both physically and mentally. I knew it: this guy was going to make it big time. I was 100 per cent sure – no, make that 100,000 per cent! Anyone could see it. The way he walked, the way he kicked a ball – one in a million was our Clarence.

Mark was ahead of his years too. So I wasn't surprised that, later on, he conquered the world with PSV, Barcelona, Bayern Munich and AC Milan. The guy won titles in Holland, Spain, Germany and Italy! All thanks to his character. Mark really lived for his sport. He was dead serious, always. Never went on the piss. His mind was always set on football. The perfect prof. Never met anyone like him.

He was the best player to come out of Limburg. Playing at number 10, as Jari Litmanen did with Ajax, nobody could get near him. Later in his career he moved towards the back of the field. That's where and how he became a superstar. But initially he was up front, with his curly hair and juvenile moustache. With his length and strength he brought us victory – more than once.

And I know it may sound strange for those of you who are familiar with his career, but in the early years he never kicked an opponent. On the contrary: at Fortuna he was always on the wrong end of the studs. He was never vengeful after being kicked, because he knew there was somebody who would do that for him.

Yup, that Ricksen guy.

I always took revenge on Mark's behalf. More than once this habit had me suspended, but I didn't care. It was all part of the deal.

For Mark this was an ideal situation. I used to 'correct' those thugs so bloody hard that they thought twice before they touched Mark again, and this meant he was free to do what he did best: playing football fluently. In this way, something nice came out of most of my passes to him.

The two of us became like a well-oiled machine. He was the artist; I was the labourer. My job in the shadows was to make him shine. It was as simple as that. And I liked it that way. It was how, in the past, a man like Jan Wouters always operated next to key figures such as Marco van Basten and Ruud Gullit.

Acting like that, Wouters was at his best. And so was I.

THREE

BREAKTHROUGH

I COULDN'T BELIEVE MY eyes. Those birds over there, in the lobby of our hotel in Bucharest, were they . . . hookers?

Of course, I'd seen a working girl before. But those women were different. More gorgeous. Hotter. Juicier. They didn't make 'em like that, back in Limburg. Oh no.

I was in Romania with the under-21s, to play in the European Championships. But despite my determination to get a good result in the pending match against the host country, football didn't seem to be that important any more. I couldn't get my eyes off those typically Eastern European girls in the corner: blonde, tall, perfectly formed and breathtakingly beautiful, and wearing practically nothing but a belt.

Irresistible!

Yes, they were whores. Why else would they be in that lobby, scantily clad and winking at everything with a dick? They were at work, simple as that.

I thought I would go mad. And, no, of course I didn't think about it! I mean, I was barely an adult. And besides, I was representing my country. If I had dragged one of those high-heeled supermodels into my room – purely hypothetical of course! – there would definitely be some punishment from the football association.

Still, I was fascinated, to put it mildly. I'd never seen prostitutes as attractive as them. And it was also the first time I'd encountered whores in a hotel lobby. I found it exciting. Maybe it was because, unlike the other guys who lived in Amsterdam, Rotterdam and Eindhoven, I was more or less a country boy. And therefore pretty naive. My teammates who played for Ajax, Feyenoord and PSV must have been familiar with drop-dead-gorgeous working girls. Yes, that must have been the case, because they didn't blink an eye while shuffling through the hotel. I, on the other hand, couldn't stop staring at those women. No penny for my thoughts!

It was 1998, and I was one of the very few players from a small club who had made it into a national team. It had been like that since 1991, when I was invited to come to the woods near the village of Zeist, where the Dutch football association has its headquarters. Me and 49 other talented kids had to show their skills on one of the FA's perfectly trimmed pitches. Each one of us had the same dream. It was just too bad there were only 31 available places.

The idea was simple: show the scouts and coaches you were good enough to become one of the chosen 31, who, after that, would have to compete for one of the eighteen orange shirts in the final squad.

And I did lay my hands on one of those jerseys. To give you an indication of the strength of this particular under-16s group, my teammates had names like Clarence Seedorf, Patrick Kluivert, Nordin Wooter, Denny Landzaat and Boudewijn Zenden (or 'Bolo', as he would be called at Chelsea, Middlesbrough, Liverpool and Sunderland). Not a bad team, eh?

Being called one of the country's best footballers in your age group is something special. Of course it is. Only I wasn't impressed at the time because I had that knowledge already. I didn't need a football association to tell me how good I was. I could pinch a ball off an opponent, I was fast, I knew a trick or two, my oversight was perfect: in short(s) I had everything it takes to be a good, modern professional football player.

Some guys have it; others don't. I had it, and I knew it.

Yet I almost missed the boat, thanks to some of my 'colleagues'. In the final, crucial match, guys from Ajax and PSV – I'm not going to mention names here, or did I do that already? – refused to pass me the ball. Why? Because doing so meant my chances of being chosen were limited. They wanted to have as many of their own in the final squad. My mother is my witness. She heard Louis van Gaal, head coach at Ajax, mentioning this strategy and even captured the quote on video.

Personally I didn't experience it quite like that. Okay, I noticed that I received the ball less than normal, but I didn't think anything bad about it. But my mother did, and, more important, Rinus Israël did too. The former Feyenoord legend, the first Dutch player ever to lift a European Cup (in 1970, after beating Celtic), was one of the men who had to judge us, together with the likes of Dick Advocaat and Bert van Lingen. Israël, one of the original Hard Men in Dutch football (nickname 'Iron Rinus'), was furious. He even ran on to the pitch and stopped the game. Anyone, he screamed in his distinctive Amsterdam accent, who in the remaining minutes of the match continued to neglect 'that little blond boy from Limburg' could pick up his gear and go home.

It worked, as the iron one wasn't somebody to mess with. About a minute later Clarence Seedorf passed me the ball. I steamed up to the box and produced a lovely pass, which Patrick Kluivert used for one of his effective headers.

I winked at Israël and Advocaat, because I knew I had made it. Fernando Ricksen was here to stay.

Immediately after that last game, I was invited by Bert van Lingen to join his juvenile squad. My mother captured the moment on camera. It was a bit of a lousy pic – sorry, Mum! – but you could still make me out, that little brat from Roda JC, and, among others, the famous Dick Advocaat from the Dutch football association.

It was the beginning of a long and beautiful period, in which one invitation for an international match after the other landed on the doormat of our humble abode. It happened so often I wasn't even surprised any more to find yet another brown FA envelope when I returned home. It was just the letters themselves that puzzled me. They always started with 'Dear sport friend'.

Sport friend? As if it was your school inviting you to a day of gymnastics!

Apart from the fame and pleasure, those international games had another advantage: they were lucrative. We didn't earn any money yet, but at least we had our expenses reimbursed. You know, petrol money and stuff. At least fifty guilders per session. That was the advantage of living so far away from Zeist. Players who had to travel from nearby Amsterdam received a lot less.

Four years later I bumped into Rinus Israël at the prestigious Festival des Espoirs youth tournament in the French city of Toulon. All of a sudden he was there, as a substitute for Hans Dorjee who couldn't be there because Guus Hiddink had chosen him to be his assistant during Euro '96 in England. Nice for Dorjee, but not so pleasant for us. For, despite his efforts to give me a fair chance four years earlier, I found him to be a weird man. Always, always negative, and a pretty crappy coach too. He couldn't even remember your name!

That led to some embarrassing situations – for him. At a point during the opening game against Russia (1–3), he wanted to give me some instructions. But all that came out of his mouth, together with some gobs of phlegm, was: 'Hey! Hey! What's your name again?'

Not very professional, eh? As an official national coach you should know who you're dealing with, even if he is 'just a little boy from Fortuna Sittard'. I thought this was all due to a lack of respect towards us. So that's why I didn't listen to him. First do your homework, Mr.

Another coach I worked with in those early years was Bert van Lingen. Now *he* was a proper coach! World class. Knew everything about everyone and was a master in building an organisation. He's the architect of the youth education department of the Dutch FA, which is considered one of the best in the world. I'm glad I met him again later on in my career, as Dick Advocaat's loyal deputy sheriff at Glasgow Rangers and Zenit Saint Petersburg.

Another top bloke in those days was Carel Akemann, the Dutch FA's jack-of-all-trades. He did *everything* for us – and I mean everything. I'm sure I must have driven him insane, as I'd always lose my money or my passport. But he always managed to solve the problem.

Despite his age – he was a pensioner already – he acted like one of the boys. When it came to topics like booze and sex, he talked like he was seventeen! And he never failed to surprise us. I remember a game against England, early 1994, which he was watching from the dug-out. Now, picture this. Second half: a ball flies through the sky like a comet, about to go way over the sideline. The old man gets up, eyes focused on the object, and . . . I swear to you, before the ball could touch the ground, it dropped dead on Mr Akemann's knee.

I was in stitches. To see the old geezer performing this Maradona-like trick, out of the blue, was an amazing sight. When he finally left the Dutch FA in 1995, after thirty years of good work – including jobs during the highly successful World Cups of 1974 and 1978 plus the triumphant Euro 1988 – I was convinced I would never forget him. His inclusion in this book proves that I was right.

Hans Dorjee was another man I fondly remember. This national youth squad coach was one of the sweetest men you'd ever meet. Never got angry, not even after a defeat. That's why we really wanted to battle for him, although it never led to grabbing a big prize, not even during that tournament in Romania. Unbelievable, given the fact that we had a squad with guys like George Boateng, Nordin Wooter, Kiki Musampa, Mario Melchiot, Arnold Bruggink, Roy Makaay and Ruud van Nistelrooy! Bronze was all we won with that dream team, would you believe it?

Poor Hans Dorjee, who sadly died in 2002 during an innocent game of tennis, wasn't to blame for this. I was. Well, sort of . . .

In the semi-final against Greece, I was rewarded with a red card, although I still object to that decision. Yes, it was a strong tackle. Yes, it was a tackle from behind. But, come on, I was kicking the ball, not the player! It just so happened that in those days referees had been given new rules. Any tackle from behind meant an automatic red card. I think the whistleblower, Miroslav Radoman, wanted to be the best student in the class, knowing UEFA and FIFA were watching him. So, yes, according to the new rules he was right, but how about a little bit of humanity? Because all of this happened *in the first minute of the game*!

So we were down to ten men for the remaining 89 minutes. And we lost. Of course we lost! 0–3.

Although I was pissed off, I still have to say that one of the Greek goals was more than just a beauty. Future Ajax and Feyenoord forward Angelos Charisteas, who would end up scoring the winning goal in the Euro 2004 final six years later, scored from almost behind the goal, with the outside of his left foot. Never seen anything like it. Our Angelos may have looked like a wooden puppet but he was one hell of a footballer. Too bad he had a Greek passport, instead of a Dutch one.

Charisteas wasn't the only youngster who I shared a pitch with who would turn out to be a superstar. There was that Portuguese bloke, Nuno Gomes. Kicked us out of the under-19s European tournament in Spain, 1994, with what can only be described as a cannonball. And then there was that French dude, a left-winger, who basically played like a machine. With or without the ball, this guy was so bloody fast! And he did practically everything right. Too bad for him his direct opponent was one Fernando Ricksen from Limburg. I sank my teeth into him from the first minute onwards – not literally of course! – and didn't give him one millimetre of space. In the end we won (3–2, thanks to two goals from Zenden and one from Kluivert), so my man hadn't been able to make the difference. But, boy, it had been a difficult evening! Out of curiosity I kept an eye on his career. And I must say I wasn't surprised to see him becoming one of the best players the English Premier League ever had. I salute you, Thierry Henry!

Still, there was an even mightier player in my younger years, despite the fact that he was tiny and prematurely balding: Ivan de la Pena. He'd never reach further than the ranks of Lazio and Espanyol, but in those early days he was the best of the lot. It was him and not so much the team who beat us 2–5 during that competition in Spain, in 1994.

We were given a chance for revenge against the Spaniards, in the so-called 'consolation final' for the third spot. Well, my teammates were offered that possibility, more to the point. I was suspended. Story of my life – already!

Yes, I was a tough guy. Whacked the odd pair of legs, and whether they belonged to an opponent or to one of our own players it was all the same to me. I didn't do it for fun, by the way, but only when I felt a little correction was required. Like, for instance, when somebody had been so unfriendly to tackle me from behind, with two legs. Not to me, buddy!

Richard Sneekes can confirm this. Still no idea what the curly-headed Sneekes (who would end up playing for Bolton Wanderers, West Bromwich Albion, Stockport County and Hull City) was thinking, that afternoon in 1993, on the training ground of Fortuna Sittard. We were just in the middle of a little position game. No tension whatsoever. Just a bit of passing the ball around and stuff. So I didn't see it coming. I only felt it.

The guy almost kicked me in two. I was crying my lungs out. What a moron! And the same goes for our coach Chris Dekker, incidentally, who didn't even stop the training.

From a distance, Mark van Bommel looked at me. He smiled. I smiled too. We both knew what was coming. In a few minutes Richard Sneekes would be dead meat. And I was the butcher.

I didn't give a toss about the fact that this poodle was only sixteen years old. I couldn't have cared less that he was about to have a beautiful career move to a foreign club. You don't try to cripple Fernando Ricksen. And if you do, you'll pay for it.

So the next moment Sneekes asked for the ball – he always asked for it, he loved the thing – I scrutinised him. And the moment he got it, I went on the attack. With two legs, just as he had done to me. I went straight for his ankles, and the noise must have been heard all the way across the border in Germany.

Game over for Richard Sneekes.

Coach Dekker was fuming. 'Fernando, what the hell? You're not gonna . . . I mean . . . one of *your own* teammates!'

'Well, he did it to me too!' I replied. 'So, better tell the little boy to stop crying. He got what he asked for.'

'*Shut your fucking mouth!*' Dekker roared.

In the corner of my eye, I could see Sneekes leaving the pitch. For a moment I was scared that I'd really seriously injured him.

Yet Richard never got angry with me. Respect! Shows that underneath all that hair, there was a top bloke. And he managed to have a nice career after all.

The fact that Mark van Bommel, who is one year younger than me, was grinning on that particular afternoon didn't surprise me. We were mates. Did our homework together, shared rooms on training camps, that kind of thing. He was a lot more serious than the rest of the guys. Mark never joined us when we sneaked out to go into town. He didn't care much about girls either. Especially not after he met Andra, daughter of the future head coach of the Dutch national team, Bert van Marwijk.

Although we were friends, I was completely different from Mark. Any chance to go out, I took it. Always. Like when we were in the Dutch seaside town of Vlissingen, at a training camp with the under-18s. I loved those camps. They gave me the opportunity to score both on and off the field. And it came easily to me, I have to confess. Girls like a good-looking football player.

So, back to the hotel it was one night, with the bird of my choice. Didn't have a clue what her name was. I was about to have a bit of carnal pleasure, and that was what counted. There was only one small problem. Mark!

Because he'd gone to bed early, being the serious guy that he was, the chick and I didn't have the room to ourselves. And, frankly, I didn't like the idea of Mark van Bommel on the sideline watching me penetrate her operational zone. I left her standing in the corridor while I woke up my pal. Would he mind leaving the room for, er, a little while so that I could play my much anticipated game of hide the sausage?

And off he went without a grumble. A true friend.

'Thanks a lot, buddy. It won't take long.'

But it did. I was simply too drunk to . . . well, you know the old Dead Kennedys song.

After an hour Mark started banging on the door, the door next to ours, to be precise. Could he sleep there 'until Fernando has finished what he has to do?'

'No,' said future Feyenoord and PSV star Patrick Paauwe. 'We don't have enough room in here.'

Of course they didn't. Both Paauwe and Vitesse's Jochem van der Hoeven were sharing the bedsheets with a girl of their own!

So, all poor Mark could do was snuggle down on a bench in the corridor. No problem for him, and we could hardly wake him up once we'd finished our business!

It wasn't just the national team that gave me the opportunity to travel – even with modest Fortuna we went away on a regular basis. In the summer of 1993 we even had a trip to China lined up. I was excited, as this was going to be my first proper flight. Fifteen hours on a plane: I was looking forward to it, believe it or not!

But it was weird. I mean, we had to go to the other side of the globe to play some kind of a tournament with . . . Roda JC, FC Utrecht and FC Twente!

Why there? Why couldn't we face them just around the corner?

Money, obviously. By running around on Chinese turf, the club would be rewarded with 150,000 guilders – plus another 50,000 for each team that would make it to the final.

So off we went. We were, after all, Fortuna Sittard, not Ajax. We needed that money.

Hey, I was going to China! It was a brilliant opportunity for a boy my age. So when I got the phone call – at, of all places, the Hommelheide campsite in Susteren where I was spending my holidays – I said yes immediately.

Hang on, you're probably thinking. No Lake Garda holiday? Yup. We'd swapped our regular Italian holiday spot for something closer to home – much closer to home! – because as a youth player at Fortuna I had to start preparations for a fresh season quite early. From 1992 onwards, six weeks in Italy was out of the question.

So our new holiday destination was Susteren, a tiny little village near the Belgian border. It was fine. I remember building myself a little wooden chalet, next to our caravan. It had a bed and a TV set inside, and on the outside a darts board. Never a dull moment.

After our stint in Susteren, my parents moved on to a campsite in Germany, a two-hour drive from the border. I didn't join them any more. Because it was too far from Sittard? No, because it wasn't far *enough*! I had caught the travellers' bug once I started moving around with my team, and I never got over it. I still love hanging around at airports and in hotel lobbies, watching the world go by.

By the way, the China trip was a disaster. Not just for us, but for all the Dutch clubs. Take the guys from Twente and Utrecht. They ate some dodgy veg and had suspicious ice cubes in their Coke. Most of them ended up as sick as a dog. Diarrhoea galore!

Basically, the only thing that stayed inside was the Roda JC squad. Inside the Phoenix hotel, that is. They were not allowed to leave it, not even to train. They were held hostage!

This was all due to Vitesse, another Dutch team who had been invited to the tournament but bottled it at the last moment, just like the Belgian clubs Liege, Bruges and Beveren. They didn't trust the organising committee and decided to stay at home.

The Chinese were pissed off, to put it mildly, not least because they had already printed lots of posters announcing the arrival of 'the best football team in the Netherlands'. They meant Vitesse.

Well, they were Chinese and no one had the internet yet.

Anyway, the sports committee in Dalian, the city that would host half of the matches, wanted to see either Vitesse or a compensatory amount of cash. Hence the fact that Roda were kept indoors, as some kind of pledge.

This was totally unacceptable to us. So, together with Utrecht and Twente, we made it clear that we wouldn't play a single minute until Roda were released. Either they let them go, or they could say 'Zai jian' to their tournament!

Oh, and we also threatened to pay a visit to the embassy.

The next morning Roda JC were free to go – from Dalian to

Shenyang, that is, some 500 kilometres down the road, where they were expected to play. It was a nice moment, also for the folks back home who had been worried.

More unusual things happened during that trip. There's the tale of Jacques Opgenoord and Pierre Schmeitz who had booked a minivan for the trip to the stadium. Halfway there, they were stopped by a policeman who confiscated the vehicle. The next moment this copper, the driver and two of Fortuna's board members were racing through the streets of Shenyang, trying to catch a truck driver who had been speeding. In doing so, they almost reduced some cyclist to a portion of satay.

The stadium in which we had to play held 70,000 spectators. And it was brand new – or so they said. 'Only one year old, sirs.'

In fact, the building looked like Rome's Colosseum. And it was dusty. So was the food. I remember the hard-boiled egg that our assistant coach Dick 'Cooky' Voorn peeled. It was black! And big. Way too big to have come out of a chicken, if you ask me.

So instead, we ate Mars bars.

No way were we eating the local food. The burgers, for instance, were stone cold. Frozen! The rice was cold too – and home to the Bacillus family. Nevertheless, the Chinese ate it by the bowlful and, even weirder, seemed to enjoy it!

Because a diet of Mars bars gets boring after a while, we decided to be polite guests in the end. On the last day we did eat some of the food. And the rest of the trip was spent on the toilet.

After twelve days we were happy to fly back home. And strange things continued to happen – even during the flight! At some stage, somewhere between Beijing and Shenyang, we had to turn back. No idea why – none of us spoke a word of Chinese – but judging by the pale, anxious faces of our fellow passengers something was terribly wrong. And damn right something was wrong: the reason we had to abandon the flight was due to an open door!

Anyway, after landing in Holland, many hours later, we made a unanimous decision: none of us would ever go back to China and we'd never eat Chinese food again.

And, as it goes, Fortuna never received all of the money. Just a lousy 50,000 guilders.

Worst of all was the fact that many of our players came back with injuries. At least seven of us were unable to play; among them our goalkeeper Ruud Hesp who had damaged his little finger.

Me, I was only shitting non-stop. No broken bones or pulled muscles, nothing. I was one of the last men standing. In international football, only the strong survive, and the ill-fated journey to China had proven that I was strong enough to make it.

After my oriental adventure, I was puzzled. Up to that point I had proven to be stronger and better than the rest of my age group. Then why oh why didn't headmaster Chris Dekker give me any credit for it? Did he really still think I wasn't good enough for the main team? I had no idea; he never spoke to me.

Come Friday, 1 October 1993, and the blackboard with the selection for the next match: the names of those who were going to face NEC in De Goffert, that ugly concrete stadium in Nijmegen. Among those names was, yes, Fernando Ricksen.

I pinched myself and had another look. It was still there.

Fernando Ricksen.

So the bugger must have changed his mind. All of a sudden I was good enough to play in Fortuna's first team. I was one day away from my debut at the highest level!

A warm feeling crept through my body. So this must be it, I said to myself. This is the feeling they always talk about. What was it they called it again? Oh yes – nerves.

I was positioned as a midfielder, on the right side, one line before René Maessen who they used to call 'Mr Fortuna'. A great honour! But it also meant that it was going to be a difficult afternoon. You see, Mr Fortuna had a habit of steaming ahead towards the opponents' box, even though he was a defender. This meant that I had to keep an eye on his spot, in case he wasn't able to return in time. So I knew I was going to make a lot of miles that afternoon.

My direct opponent would be a guy named Kees van Wonderen. Although playing for NEC in the First Division, he was already a force to be reckoned with. In a few years' time he would play for Feyenoord and the national team. You could see that coming. The guy was good. And he *never* stood still.

So with Maessen constantly running away from me and van Wonderen constantly running towards me, I was constantly on the move. At one stage I got sick of it and cursed Mr Fortuna, told him to stay on his spot once in a while. He wasn't having any of it and just kept going. And so did I, until I was totally out of breath. After an hour I had to be taken off the pitch. I couldn't even blame Dekker for my substitution. I was empty, completely empty.

Besides, I had shown I was eager and good enough for this level. So I had earned myself plenty of other chances. Or had I?

No. In the remainder of the 1993/94 season I played a few more minutes against Veendam – and that was it.

Of course, I sensed some kind of a conspiracy. The older players, in my opinion, were scared of me. They thought I was better than them, so I had to be kept out of the team. That's why they never helped me at all. Same with Mark, who debuted a few months before me, against Cambuur Leeuwarden. They didn't like his skills either. Luckily Mark and I had each other. Without his support, I may well have drowned. Who knows? It's a strange world, professional football. I always thought of it as a team sport; you know, togetherness and solidarity. I was wrong.

We ended in tenth place that season, with just 33 points from 34 games. So Chris Dekker had to leave. No chemistry any more, as they say.

Enter Pim Verbeek, a former Feyenoord coach. His task: bring Fortuna Sittard back to the Eredivisie, the Dutch Premier League. Ambition at last! I was totally up for it, but we had a bit of a problem. Verbeek said I was a defender, not a midfielder. But that spot, on the right side of the field, belonged to René Maessen. Actually, it had been his spot for sixteen long seasons, so when I say he was already playing there when I was still in nappies, I am not exaggerating! Besides, he was doing well. There was no need at all to have him replaced by that young kid Ricksen.

Here we go again, I thought. One available spot and it belongs to a guy who has played more than 400 games in that position. What to do?

Training, as hard and intense as possible. That's all I could do. Hope he would break his legs? No way. First, if I wanted to reach the top, I had to do it with my own ability; that was my idea. Second, Maessen was a nice guy. Simple as that.

Eventually Maessen *did* lose his spot to me. It was just after an under-19s tournament in Spain that I made my way into the first XI – for 30 matches. Now, Maessen could have been extremely pissed off with that, but he wasn't. He wished me, his successor, the best of luck and even helped me here and there. Now that's what I call a good teammate!

And what a year we had! Due to a 2–0 victory at Telstar on the last day of the season – 13 May 1995 – we won the title in the First Division, ending up with just one point more than our main rivals, De Graafschap. Back on the highest level at last!

All credit to Pim Verbeek for giving youngsters like Mark van Bommel, Maurice Rayer, Roberto Lanckohr and, er, me a fair chance. The average age of our wonder team was 22, so that more or less sums it up. The celebrations in the town centre of Sittard were massive. We had thousands of fans singing to us on the main market square – at one-thirty in the morning! All you could hear was 'Fortuna noa veure!', authentic Limburgian for 'Go, Fortuna, go!' Nobody was thinking about the bonus of 220,000 guilders we would receive after winning the title. Who cared? After all, it was 220,000 divided by 22 players.

From that moment on, I got better and better, stronger and stronger. None of the big guys, whether they played for Ajax, Feyenoord or PSV, could mess with me. I became a 'better than average' player in the Dutch League simply by standing my ground.

Until a fateful moment in 1995, just before Christmas, when I became the man who fell to earth – literally – after an unlucky slide by PSV's Ernest Faber on a frozen pitch (it was minus seven that day) in Eindhoven. I fell and I couldn't get back up. My ankle hurt like hell and I was in a lot of pain. I thought it was the end of my career.

The next day, in hospital, it was revealed that I had torn ligaments in three different places. Well, it was Crimbo time, so I wouldn't miss *that* many games. A few weeks in plaster and I would make my comeback. I was convinced of it. And indeed, on 24 February, ten weeks after the collision, I was kicking a ball again, in an away game against Sparta. The doctor said it was close to a miracle, the fastest recovery he'd ever seen.

Nevertheless, that ankle became my weak spot. My Achilles' heel. Much later, at Rangers and at Zenit, it happened more than once that I had to stay on the bench. Too much pain. Still, that rehabilitation period taught me how to fight properly. Those were the weeks in which I developed my so-called fighting spirit. Battling pain that was cutting through my body like a hot knife, day in, day out, was hell, but I had to do it. I didn't want to run away from it. Couldn't run away from it. I was challenging demons, provoking them, only to be rewarded with the most acute pain I'd ever felt in my entire life. But I had to do it in order to get stronger. I had to come to terms with the limitations of my body and expand them.

The reward for my efforts came in 1997, when I won one of the most valuable individual prizes in Dutch football. I became Rookie of the Year, as chosen by the editors and reporters of leading Dutch football weekly *Voetbal International*. I was ahead of guys like Jon Dahl Tomasson, Boudewijn Zenden, Mario Melchiot and George Boateng, to name a few. And, to make things even better, the prize was given to me by none other than the mighty Johan Cruyff.

So, in order not to look like a provincial jerk, I bought some new clothes for the occasion: a white shirt with a black, sleeveless leather waistcoat. It was the nineties, okay? And, yes, it did make me look like a provincial jerk.

'If you continue like this,' Cruyff told me, 'you have a great future ahead of you.' I think I nodded, or maybe I said yes. Definitely no more than that. For this was the one and only Johan Cruyff, the greatest Dutch footballer of all time. And in the presence of someone like Cruyff, even Fernando Ricksen is quiet.

Oh, and I got a pair of new boots! Cruyff Sports, naturally. Well known in Amsterdam, but a novelty in Limburg, where everybody was wearing Puma or adidas. With my pair of Cruyff shuffles, I was The Man, feet-wise.

Too bad they only lasted for a few weeks.

FOUR

THE WILD WEST

IN THE SPRING OF 1997 I was on the up, thanks to my excellent performances at Fortuna Sittard and 'Young Orange'. According to the press, clubs were even lining up to sign me. And we're talking about the likes of Liverpool, Borussia Dortmund and Bayer Leverkusen here! It was the 'air' of this snotty kid from Limburg, as one reporter put it. He was referring to my, well, not arrogance, but . . . self-confidence. I think that's the word. And as much as I had seen this coming, I enjoyed every minute of it. Even Pim Verbeek admitted that I was ready for a big jump forward. He called me a 'total player' meaning you could use me anywhere on the pitch. And I never let myself nor my team down. The least I scored on a weekly basis was seven out of ten.

I kinda liked the guy. Good man, Verbeek. He always treated me with respect and, more important, really wanted the best for me. 'If the big clubs are coming to sign him, we won't keep him here,' I once heard him say. He refused to tell me that staying at Fortuna for one more year would be the best thing to do, in terms of my development, because he knew it was complete bullshit. And I agreed.

Anyway, the word 'bullshit' also sums up the alleged line of clubs that was out there, just waiting to sign me. I never received an official offer. In the end I had to come to terms with the fact that it had all been rumour.

The only club that really, really wanted me was AZ Alkmaar. And they'd just been relegated . . . No way, I thought initially. Fortuna were playing in the League; why would I want to change that for a season in the First Division? And what about the national team? They wouldn't be interested in a footballer who wasn't even playing in the country's major competition!

Come July, I had signed for AZ. For five seasons.

No, I wasn't nuts. The club was owned by one Dirk Scheringa, a banker who was burning with ambition. 'We're gonna create something big in Alkmaar,' he said, at the headquarters of his DSB bank in the tiny village of Wognum, north of Amsterdam. As much as I was an up-and-coming player, DSB was an up-and-coming bank, trying to rub shoulders with the likes of ABN-Amro and ING.

'Within three years,' he said, as the traffic of the A7 motorway sped past the building, 'I want AZ to be part of the League's top three. And I need you to realise those plans.'

I was flattered. Always nice to get the occasional bit of appreciation!

'Within five years, I want AZ to win the League,' he continued. That, he revealed, was his ultimate goal, his dream: breaking the supremacy of Ajax, Feyenoord and PSV. Unreal? No, it had happened before, in 1981. So why not again?

I liked his dream, but at the same time I thought: cheese capital Alkmaar is pretty far away from the trusted hills of Limburg. He noticed my reservation, and played his next card, designed to convince me to sign for AZ. He started mentioning the names of players he wanted to sign or already had signed: guys like Barry van Galen, Michel Langerak, Peter van den Berg and Robert van der Weert. Each of them was too good for the First Division. I liked it.

Apart from them, I was told, the club had contracted the extremely talented goalkeeper Oscar Moens, as well as Kenneth Perez and Dries Boussatta. Plus John Bosman of Ajax and Orange fame.

'Oh, and we want to pay you half a million a year.' He said it just like that. As if he was ordering a sandwich. And, if I decided to sign for five seasons, I would get a brand new Audi TT.

I was glowing. One scribble and I would be the owner of the latest top-of-the-range Audi. And with it came this enormous amount of money.

I started to calculate. Five times half a million guilders is . . . Two! And! A! Half! Million! Excluding bonuses. I would be a millionaire!

I had to sign. Big deal that he couldn't tell me the name of the new coach yet. The future looked brighter than bright. And with AZ at the top of the League, there was a big chance that I would make my debut in the national team before the tender age of 25, just as I had predicted!

Fortuna paid me 1,500 guilders a month. At AZ I would get thirty times as much. Who would think twice in a situation like that?

I never thought much of players who insisted that money doesn't matter. I found them hypocritical. What was wrong with admitting that you liked to earn a shitload? I'd always said that I wanted to be financially independent before turning 30. A professional football player has only a limited number of years to get wealthy. You better use that short period well.

Fortuna hit the jackpot too. Because I had signed for three years AZ had to buy me out. I think my old club received 1.5 million guilders for me. Fortuna – what an appropriate name!

I liked joining AZ, but wasn't too smitten with the town of Alkmaar. As some of us know, citizens and tourists, they sell cheese over there, in a market square. Well, good luck to them. I was only interested in training and playing games. Even when my parents came to visit me, we never went into town. We always drove to Amsterdam, which has a lot more to offer. I didn't mind acting like a tourist over there. Oh no, the three of us even jumped in one of those canal boats to look at all the old buildings.

Talking about old buildings: AZ's stadium, the 'Alkmaarderhout', was falling apart, a complete mess. Farmers wouldn't let their cattle graze in such a dismal environment! It was just a matter of time, Scheringa told me. I had to be patient. Within years the club would be the proud owner of one of the most modern stadiums in the country. 'Other clubs will envy us, Fernando,' he said with a smile. 'We just have to wait for the right permits, but once we have them . . .'

He didn't need to finish his sentence. Playing for AZ, the ultimate challenge in Dutch football, I loved it already!

I got a house in Callantsoog, a seaside resort twenty minutes' drive west of Alkmaar. This was thanks to Hugo Hovenkamp, a former player from the Golden AZ of the early eighties (the one that won the title and played the UEFA Cup Final against Ipswich Town). Hovenkamp had some property there, so it was easy for me and Esther, my puppy love from Limburg, to move in.

To me, this was an ideal situation. I lived next to the sea, which is a perfect spot for a player to concentrate on the next game. After a training session, I often went to the beach to do some running. I was totally living for my sport. Jogging on the beach had completely replaced my old pattern of going down the pub. I was a different person now – and I liked it. All the boozing and chasing birds – I didn't care any more. I became a couch potato. Watching TV with Esther, you get the picture. Yup, it might sound boring, but I felt great. And so did she. We loved each other's company, and basically that was all that mattered to us. And why would I risk this perfect little life with my sweetheart with bad behaviour?

However, things would change within two years, after we moved to the centre of Alkmaar. Esther got homesick and wanted to go back to Sittard. I couldn't stop her. If I did, it would be a lose/lose situation.

I went to Alkmaar because, to be honest, I did get a bit bored with the quietness of Callantsoog. At least Alkmaar was a little more exciting. That's what I heard from the boys in the dressing room. They went out for a drink or two and always ended up with some extra fun, because they were players from the local football club. All of a sudden running on the beach and watching TV seemed extremely dull to me. I wanted to rejoin the circus!

So I started on a little pub crawl now and then, most of the time accompanied by guys I knew from the gym. Freefighters.

Interesting guys. I could relate to them. And, more important, they respected me.

Pretty soon, we changed our hunting turf and went to Amsterdam instead. In fact, we did it so often that I became a regular at the Cooldown Café, a notorious party pub at Rembrandtplein, one of the city's main entertainment squares. The poison of choice over there: shots. Lots of them. Because I still lived for my sport, we avoided the weekends and went out on a Monday. Traditionally that's the evening on which barkeepers and pub owners themselves go out to quench their thirst.

Unlike in Alkmaar – or Sittard, for that matter – you always met a lot of famous people in Amsterdam. Sports presenters, actors, that kind of thing. And actresses, of course. I remember bumping into a chick who had just started playing in the soap opera *Goede Tijden, Slechte Tijden* ('Good Times, Bad Times'), Holland's very own *EastEnders*. And, yes, I spent the night with her.

My freefighter friends also took me to kickboxing events. We always had the best tickets, so I was only a few inches away from the most beautiful uppercuts and low kicks. I absolutely loved it! Needless to say I tried to do a bit of it myself too, at the gym, but I'd always be aware of the dangers. So I took it easy. And asked the others to take it easy on me.

It was in those days that Pedro and my parents noticed a bit of a change in my character. They were right, but I didn't notice it myself. I was way too self-centred for that. 'Tunnel vision' might best describe it. At one stage, I didn't even bother talking to them any more.

Despite the partying, I was still delivering the goods when it came to playing football. My stats: 31 games in my second season, 29 in the third. A pisshead couldn't have achieved that! To be honest, I never drank that much in those days. Sometimes I didn't even consume a single drop of alcohol. Like, for instance, when we went to the Baja Beach Club in Rotterdam, home to the most gorgeous and largest-breasted girls this side of Hollywood. Like the women's bras, the place was always loaded – every night of the week. It was worth driving an extra hour, I can tell you! And, as most of the time I was the driver, I stuck to soft drinks. Couldn't bear the thought of being caught behind the wheel with alcohol running through my veins, or, worse, causing an accident. That would be the end of my career, no doubt about it.

And let's face it: when it came to football I had it all, at that very moment. A great contract with a very ambitious club, good results and a future so bright I had to wear shades. It was perfect! No way was I going to put that at risk for a few beers!

The fact that I was doing so well at AZ was largely thanks to my first coach over there, Willem van Hanegem. We're talking about the legendary De Kromme ('The Crooked One') here, the man who won the European Cup and World Cup for Clubs (both 1970) as well as the UEFA Cup (1974) with Feyenoord, and who, according to Brian Glanville, was the best player of the lot at the World Cup tournament of 1974. He was a legend, living a life totally devoted to football. We immediately hit it off.

He helped me whenever he could, made me better than I already was. And not just me, he did it with everyone! A genius, Willem van Hanegem. And a brilliant comedian too. Sarcastic, cynical, dry. Not everyone's cup of tea, but I loved it.

One day, during a pre-match talk, he said, 'You better perform tonight, guys. Apart from being rewarded with a nice bag of cash, the most beautiful girls will be lining up for you. Chicks want winners, no matter how ugly those winners are. With good results on the pitch, even a rotten corpse like Dennis can get lucky.' And with that, he pointed at our teammate Dennis den Turk.

Everybody was in stitches, while Dennis looked like he could eat the coach and spit him out, there and then. But there were no real hard feelings. Next time, somebody else would be on the receiving end. And then Dennis would laugh, just as much as the others. It was Van Hanegem's unique interpretation of the team-building concept. And it worked. We finished our first season as champions, seven points ahead of the number two, Cambuur Leeuwarden. Back into the League we went! AZ were ready to challenge Ajax,

Feyenoord and PSV, just as Dirk Scheringa had predicted. Well, all credit to Willem van Hanegem, a superb coach!

But it wasn't all sunshine. At times, Van Hanegem could be grumpy – very grumpy. Like that day in December 1998 when he entered our dressing room after we'd just beaten Roda JC. He had a face like thunder. So we were expecting a tirade. Especially me, because in the match I had received a red card after flooring Marc Nygaard.

But it wasn't about me. He had a surprise for all of us, he said. And we wouldn't like it, he predicted. The suspense!

'Boys . . .' he said, in a melodramatic voice.

Silence.

'Boys, I'm leaving.'

And off he went!

We couldn't even ask him about the reasons for his decision. He just walked out the door!

We didn't get it. Weren't we the big attraction in the Dutch League? Okay, we weren't title challengers yet, but we played some of the best and most stylish football in the country! We even managed to beat Feyenoord and PSV.

Later on, we heard there had been some kind of a hiccup between Scheringa and Van Hanegem. But the tension didn't last for long, as shortly after Van Hanegem signed for another five years – only to leave at the end of that very season.

On and off the pitch, you simply can't follow Willem van Hanegem.

Thinking about the man now, I remember him as a fanatical player on fruit machines. We didn't get a look in. He even did it between training sessions! And he had a trick to prevent others from taking over his spot, the stingy bastard. He always left one point on the slot machine, before he shuffled off to the training ground. Now, there's an unwritten law among gamblers: you don't touch a machine that still has points on it. Why did he do that? Because he was scared that someone would come and take out the money he'd been throwing in for the past hour.

Everyone knew that the single point on the flickering fruit machine belonged to our coach. So nobody dared touch the damn thing. No way, we all wanted to be on the pitch next weekend!

After Van Hanegem finally left AZ we got a new coach: Gerard van der Lem. He was a highly successful assistant to Louis van Gaal at the mighty Ajax of the nineties. Together they managed to win the UEFA Cup (1992), Champions League (1995) and Club World Cup (1995). They had joined forces at Barcelona too. AZ would be the first big job on his own, so I didn't know what to expect. A good assistant isn't always a good main man.

Well, at least Van der Lem knew a thing or two about football. To people who've never played at the highest level, his talks may have sounded like rocket science mixed with mathematics, but to me it all made sense. Everything he said was very, very interesting. And unlike Van Hanegem, Van der Lem really had a vision for the future. Perfect! And he was always on your side, never on the side of the club. Loved that! So the inevitable happened: under Van der Lem I would have my best season at AZ. As a right midfield player I even started to score again: nine times in total. I was doing so well I was even close to the final squad for Euro 2000. Sadly, together with guys like Patrick Paauwe, Michel Kreek and Orlando Trustfull, I didn't make it to the final stages. A real pity, as the tournament was to be held in our own country and the national coach was none other than the legendary Frank Rijkaard.

Anyway, this near-selection was telling me I was on the right path. And I was: more and more big clubs started to show some interest in me. Like the club where Dick Advocaat was working: Glasgow Rangers.

Rangers! One of the biggest British clubs ever!

I got hot flushes, started to shake. Would AZ let me go?

'Fernando,' Van der Lem said, as I told him about the Scottish interest, 'when a club like Glasgow Rangers comes around . . .'

It felt like my heart was trying to fight its way out of my chest.

'. . . you should always do it. Always! I don't want to see you go. For AZ you're of great importance, but as an individual you can get much, much better at a club like Rangers. Besides, it's useless to keep a player against his will. I've seen that at Ajax, with Edgar Davids. Nobody wins in a situation like that.'

Thanks, Gerard, I thought. Now off to Dirk Scheringa, with the 'good news'. I wonder how he . . .

'Fifteen million guilders and not a cent less!'

Okay, clear. He wasn't going to let me go just like that. I didn't like this. I knew I was totally sane when I signed a five-year contract with AZ, but gimme a break. No disrespect to AZ, but this was, for God's sake, Glasgow fucking Rangers!

Why did Scheringa do this? There's a big, big club fishing for one of your players. That player could benefit from the catch, both financially and in terms of becoming a better sportsman. Didn't he always say I was his favourite member of the squad? Then why would he stop me in my personal development? C'mon, Mr Scheringa, please . . .

No.

Fifteen million guilders. Otherwise it would be the red shirt of AZ for a few more years, instead of the mighty blue of the Gers. I thought I was going mad.

The fact that Rangers wanted me hadn't come as a big surprise, as my former mentor, Dick Advocaat, was their head coach. I'd always seen him as a kind of father figure. I liked him, and he liked me. Maybe because in many ways, we were the same: open and honest. Apart from that, Dick had been a player like me, in his days at numerous clubs such as FC Den Haag, Roda JC, Sparta, FC Utrecht and Chicago Sting. Always fanatical, always determined to grab the ball. Always in trouble with the ref, because he never kept his mouth shut. But also: willing to do the heavy, 'dirty' work in order to let the stars of the team shine. He wanted a guy like that at Rangers. I could be that guy.

It was the end of 1999 when he called me. Was I interested in coming to Scotland?

What a stupid question, I thought. Of course I wanted to go to Scotland! Okay, as a child I had dreamed about England, Italy and Spain, but this wasn't just Scotland, it was Glasgow Rangers!

Rangers, with fans all over the world: in Asia, South America, the United States and South Africa. Name one big city in the world and I bet you they have a Glasgow Rangers supporters' club. And all of those clubs have their specific fan club days, when they're visited by players. I'm not kidding: I remember visiting one of those events in New York, 2001. Thousands of fans, thousands of miles away from Ibrox, and all dressed in blue! Eat that, PSV! They think they're a big international football club, but the only fan clubs outside their own city are located in Helmond and Mierlo. Which, for your information, are towns at a crawling distance from Eindhoven.

Laughable, really. And don't think you'll bump into someone like Sean Connery when you visit PSV v. FC Groningen. Well, at Ibrox, the original James Bond has his own throne, high above the main stand. That impressed me.

Summer of 2003, as *The League of Extraordinary Gentlemen* was showing in cinemas all over Britain, I met Sir Sean in the pub. Ronald de Boer is my witness. We had just beaten FC Copenhagen and qualified for the Champions League, so some well-earned drinks were already inside us. Ronald, bless him, walked towards Sir Sean and said, 'So you really think you can enter the Grand Canal in Venice with a submarine?'

Connery looked at us, like only he can, and said, 'Chaps, do you know how much I earned with that job?'

'No idea,' we answered.

'Seventeen million pounds,' he said, as he gave each of us a pat on the back. And off he went, smiling.

Back to that phone call in 1999. Couldn't get it out of my head. I realised that Rangers was a club at which I could win prizes. Important prizes! With Rangers I could play the Champions League. That is every single footballer's dream – and it was up for grabs! So why, why, why wouldn't AZ allow me to make this giant leap? I had done my utmost on behalf of the club in previous seasons, so why would they want to punish me?

That's exactly what I said to Scheringa. I was close to tears. 'Please, please give me this chance, after all I've done for AZ . . .'

But he wouldn't give in.

So, one day, I decided to visit him in Wognum. I wanted to make a last-ditch attempt to change his mind. Or at least change it a little bit. He was stubborn – we all knew that – but I wanted to show him how much it hurt me.

I went on my own. I didn't need any help. After all I wasn't scared of anyone, no matter how rich they might be.

As an aside: I hold no hard feelings towards Dirk Scheringa. He has done great things for Alkmaar and the area. Yes, AZ does play in a modern stadium nowadays and they did win the title in 2009. That was all thanks to Dirk. But at the same time he was a hard bastard, especially when it came to business. And it was that Scheringa I had to face, that day in Wognum.

'I do understand, Fernando,' he kept repeating. 'But this isn't entirely about you. It's about the club too – and you'll understand that, being the owner, I have to think about the club.'

In short: he wanted the maximum amount of money for me. But he didn't want to sell me at all, because he didn't want to destroy what he called 'a fantastic team'.

Yes, I understood his point of view. Of course I did. But I was pissed off too. And I thought: okay, you want to play hard, let's really play hard. So I decided to take him to court if things didn't go the way I wanted.

Together with my agent, Henk van Ginkel, I studied the possibilities. It was obvious: despite the contract, this was a matter of getting a better and more important job, an increase in status. On top of that, Rangers wanted to pay eight million for me. Not exactly the fifteen Scheringa wanted, but still an awful lot of money for a kid from Limburg.

Scheringa was not impressed.

Instead, he went on the counter-attack and offered me a contract for life. Yes, life. He'd done that already with Oscar Moens. And this, dear reader, meant a lot of money for yours truly. An awful lot of money. One million guilders a year – for a period of fifteen years. Guaranteed. And excluding bonuses.

I would be completely and totally independent, financially speaking. I just had to sign. I didn't. Nope.

Don't want your money, Mr Scheringa. I want to go to Scotland. To Glasgow. 'Paradise', according to Michael Mols who was already there. 'Don't think twice, just go!' he told me. 'Aren't you on a plane yet?'

I couldn't wait. I wanted it so badly. I wanted to play an Old Firm match more than anything else. The infamous clash between Celtic and Rangers, Catholics versus Protestants: I'd heard about it so often and it completely set my heart on fire.

The hatred between those two teams . . . Once you've played for the greens, you don't go to the blues – or vice versa. Unless you're Mo Johnston, but that's another story. Former Celtic star and fellow countryman Pierre van Hooijdonk knew what would have happened if he'd said yes to Rangers, so that's why he said no. Dick Advocaat wanted him, after Pierre's adventures in Turkey, but Pierre said no. 'Too dangerous. And out of respect for Celtic.'

Personally I couldn't care less whether I dealt with a Catholic, a Protestant or a Muslim. I was – and still am – way too down-to-earth for all that hassle. Yes, I was raised in a Catholic environment and, yes, as a kid I even went to a Catholic church. But I would still end up playing for a Protestant club like Rangers. I didn't have any problems with that at all.

The Old Firm clash just happens to be the most exciting thing in football. Ronald de Boer had warned me already: 'It's a hundred times more intense than Ajax v. Feyenoord!' And Michael Mols simply couldn't stop talking about it. So I went ballistic: I had to play an Old Firm match!

But Dirk Scheringa wasn't having any of it. According to him, I belonged to AZ. At this stage, I really got nervous. And things got worse when Ruud van Nistelrooy got injured, just as he was about to go to Manchester United. Okay, he recovered, but what if a thing like that happened to me and I stayed injured? Then it would be a matter of bye bye Rangers, nice not meeting you!

I didn't want to take the risk. But still I did. I am simply not the kind of player who 'uses the handbrakes'. I never play at 75 per cent. The fact that an injury could have been disastrous for my future didn't mean that I played super-carefully. Both in matches and in training I always wanted to win, so I always went for the ball – even during a shitty little run-around. And I still hit the odd teammate once in a while. Not on purpose, although you can't really feel the difference. Ask Barry Opdam, who I sadly mistook for the ball. I can still hear him screaming. Well, he would, wouldn't he? His shinbone was kinda battered. Industrial injury though, isn't it?

So he stayed on the grass and I walked way, like I almost always did. Through the years I've received the occasional kick too, but I can't remember ever stopping a training session because of it. You know what? I may interrupt one the moment I lose an entire leg. But not before.

But Barry, poor Barry, went to the dressing room in tears. I thought it was ridiculous. Take a sponge, wash off the blood and get on with it, please! And, no, things like this happen in professional football, so I didn't feel the urge to apologise.

My teammates totally disagreed, especially José Fortes Rodriguez. He was furious. I'd done it on purpose, he said. Well, fuck you, mate! I don't give a toss what you think. I went for a shower, got dressed and left. As I drove homeward, I wasn't even thinking about it any more. Rodriguez, on the other hand, was still talking about it five years later . . .

Oh yeah, Rodriguez. He wanted revenge for Opdam and went for me on the training ground over and over again – with the assistance of Barry van Galen, one of the hardest men in Dutch football. But they never caught me. I was simply too fast for them. At the same time I thought, if they want to play hard, I'll play hard too! As the guy in *The Incredible Hulk* used to say: 'Don't make me angry. You wouldn't like me when I'm angry!'

It was obvious that José was envious of me. He saw me getting better and better by the day. Every single thing I did with the ball went right. That stung. I knew he was trying to hurt me on purpose, I could sense it. Well, it takes one to know one.

In the beginning I liked the guy, but after a while I felt we were too different. For me, mediocrity wasn't enough. I wanted the best – and I wanted to work hard to achieve that. So going out with the guys for a coffee didn't fit in that picture. Gimme a break. Why should we socialise all the time, just because we play in the same football team?

José didn't like my attitude. He said I was selfish and didn't show any respect to the team. I thought it was hilarious. I was on my way to the top, I didn't have time for this sentimental shit. Oh, I totally understood him! After all, I was on the verge of a transfer to an international superpower, while he was and always would be a simple defender at a modest Dutch club.

Okay, I have to take this back, a little bit. José did have his qualities for the team. He was the perfect twelfth man.

His anger didn't only rotate around my being his rival on the pitch. No, things had happened off the pitch too.

Her name was Graciela. Blonde and drop-dead gorgeous. I met her in Alkmaar and pretty soon we started dating. The problem was, José wanted her too. Desperately. But Graciela, who knew him already, couldn't stand him.

So, there you go. Time to move on and leave AZ behind, for all sorts of reasons. There was way too much negativity there. So I called my agent.

'Let's go to Scotland,' I said to Henk.

'Why?'

'To negotiate.'

He knew I wasn't bullshitting. I meant it.

In the meantime Rangers had made three different offers: 10.2 million, 10.8 million and, eventually, around 13 million guilders.

Thirteen. Million. Guilders.

I thought it was a fair amount of money. More than fair, to tell you the truth. After all, at that time I hadn't played a single match for the national team. I was just a nice player at a small provincial club. So thirteen million would be . . .

'Not enough,' according to Scheringa. He still wanted his fifteen million. 'Rangers are top, you are top, so the sum should be top too,' he said.

Now I was starting to get very, very pissed off. I had no idea if AZ knew I was going to Glasgow to talk. I didn't care. I knew what I was doing was a breach of contract, but I still did it. The situation was killing me. I wanted this transfer so badly.

And then Middlesbrough made an offer too. I didn't think much of it though. Boro, with all respect, is a club you can't rely on. Premier League one year, Championship the other. No stability at all. Besides, to be selected for the Dutch national team, you had – and still have, I suppose – to play at the highest level. Boro couldn't guarantee that.

Still, it made me nervous. What if Middlesbrough wanted to pay the fifteen million? Would Scheringa sell me to them, just like that? Like a cow? I tried not to think about it too much, as the whole situation was really getting to me.

As we landed at Glasgow International Airport, it was raining. Of course it was raining, it was Scotland! But you know what? I didn't care! I like shitty weather! It allows me to play the way I want to. I'm a tough guy, remember? And as soon as I saw the stadium I knew: this was where I wanted to play.

Even at the tender age of 23 I'd seen a lot of stadiums already, but this . . . this was *it*!

The moment I walked into Edmiston Drive it was like the dark clouds vanished and the sun shone through. There it was: the mighty Ibrox Stadium!

It was love at first sight.

Fifty thousand seats. A beautiful cast-iron gate. Stained-glass windows. Where on earth did you see stained-glass windows other than in a church?

I knew it, I knew it: this is where I wanted to write history!

Inside the stadium, in the pounding heart of Rangers Football Club I felt nothing but warmth. Wherever I looked I saw ancient photos depicting the rich history of this phenomenal club. It was like being in a museum!

And at that point I hadn't even seen the Blue Room, the centuries-old boardroom. The grandeur of the place was overwhelming, especially to a kid from Little Chicago. There were beautiful armchairs swathed in red and blue, and portraits of famous people from the club's history painted by Senga Murray, wife of chairman David. I walked past them, like you do in places like the Louvre and the National Gallery, and had a good look at everything. There they all were: big shots like Graeme Souness, Andy Goram, Jim Baxter, Davie Cooper, Mark Hateley, Walter Smith, John Greig and, hey, Ally McCoist, the crafty goal machine. Yes, this club really knows how to honour its heroes!

I closed my eyes and saw an addition to the collection: Fernando Ricksen, as painted by Senga Murray. I was on cloud nine . . . Until I remembered the wooden hovel of AZ, in Alkmaar, where I was playing.

'We can't blow this!' I hissed at van Ginkel. 'Henk, we're not leaving until we have a deal!'

I was pretty confident. Henk van Ginkel was one hell of a negotiator, and I trusted him to reach an agreement. No doubt about it. The man had a card or two up his sleeve. The way he had handled my transfer to AZ three years earlier – brilliant!

Strangely enough, this time he didn't need all of his bargaining skills. The negotiating went as smoothly as the legs of my beloved Graciela. Chairman Murray agreed on everything we proposed. Before I realised it, I had an annual salary of £800,000 – once again, excluding bonuses!

I was going to earn about seven times as much as in Alkmaar. Talk about a good deal! Oh, and on top of that Rangers would provide me with free flights to Holland plus a new car, an Opel. Thanks, Mr Murray, it's highly appreciated!

If only Dirk Scheringa didn't shatter my dreams . . .

'Congratulations Fernando,' he said to me, one afternoon in March. 'Rangers and AZ have made a deal. As from next season, you'll be playing in Scotland.'

I was so over the moon I wanted to hear it again.

'As from next season you'll be playing in Scotland.'

They'd made a deal. A few weeks after my sneaky trip to Glasgow, Rangers and AZ struck a deal. The Gers decided to pay those fifteen million guilders to AZ. In the end there were only winners. Rangers were happy to have me, I was happy to go to Rangers, and Scheringa was happy to get his cash.

And maybe even José Fortes Rodriguez could be a winner, I thought with a devious smile on my face. That is, if AZ used some of the transfer money to create a new training ground . . .

FIVE

DOUBTS

BECAUSE I WAS AWARE of the – how to put this? – sensitive relationship between Celtic and Rangers, I decided to throw a bit of oil on the fire. It was my official presentation in the Ibrox press room, May 2000, and I was up for a laugh. And I got the perfect assist to score that goal; 'receiving the ball on your tie', as we say in the Netherlands. Scoring had never been so easy.

'Fernando,' one of the journos asked, 'what do you think of Celtic?'

'Celtic?' I answered with a frown. 'What's that?'

Diabolical laughter filled the room. I'd made my point. My God, those sports hacks went mad! But not because the joke had been that brilliant. No, they were completely taken aback by the fact that this newcomer had the guts to say a thing like that. Basically they were laughing the tension away. They hadn't seen that goal coming!

I could fully understand them. There aren't many things as boring as the presentation of a new player. Most of the time it's a matter of producing some prefabricated quotes such as 'I am very happy to be here', after which the new purchase puts his scribble on a piece of paper and grins in the photographers' flashlights.

Instead, I decided to put on a show – without thinking about the consequences. Typical me. I didn't realise that with one innocent little joke I had instantly made millions of enemies.

From that moment on, they hated me. And that was no joke.

According to the green hordes, I needed to be punished.

From then on, whenever I walked into a shop or just down the street, I would be verbally abused by Celtic fans. It was only then that I grasped how serious the hatred between the two clubs' supporters was.

This was unheard of in Holland. Who in Amsterdam would give a toss that I was playing for AZ? And what about Limburg, with its four professional football clubs? As a Fortuna player I had no problems at all walking the streets of Maastricht or Venlo. Locals would even wave at me.

Not so in Bonnie Scotland. Celtic fans even spat in my face. Yelling, cursing, swearing, it happened over and over again. And not just to me; Graciela was a target too. For her, all this verbal abuse took the fun out of shopping.

Most of the time we just walked on, ignoring the shouts of 'fuckers', 'wankers' and 'bastards' that buzzed around our heads like bluebottles. Not because I was scared. I was never scared. It's just that I didn't want this to turn into something major. I knew it was provocation. They wanted to see if they could annoy me enough to receive a few well-deserved whacks. That, then, would have given them the right to hit back.

I believe that their anger was fuelled by some of the scumbags of the British press. During the aforementioned press conference I had also talked about my aims and ambition at Glasgow Rangers; not a single word of that statement made it into the tabloids. Instead, all they wrote about was the 'terrible' way I had 'insulted' Celtic, and in headlines the size of doughnuts.

But it wasn't an insult, it was meant to be a bloody joke! Nobody believed me, of course. And from that moment on I was the bad guy.

Then, things got a lot worse. I wasn't just hated by Celtic fans, I was hated in the rest of Scotland too! I've no idea how they managed to get my number, but I started to receive horrible phone calls – at horrible hours.

'I know which school your child goes to.' That was about Wim, my barely ten-year-old stepson. They even called him, poor kid, and told him they would come around to 'visit' him.

A little boy. How low can you sink?

I was terrified now, but I couldn't show it. I had to be strong for Wim and Graciela. If I had shown fear they wouldn't have felt safe any more. So I acted as if I didn't care, went into everything's-fine mode, and managed to suppress my fear and my anger. Until March 2005 . . .

What happened then was beyond belief. I was checking my fan mail, like any other day. I always received lots of letters, confirmation of the fact that you're a popular player. I loved them: the requests for an autograph or a photo, the long, hand-written letters some people sent and the occasional pair of panties. Yeah, I loved my job!

But this envelope, on this specific morning, shortly before the League Cup Final against Motherwell, obviously contained something else. I noticed it the moment I took it out of my locker. This was not your average letter. And I was right: inside the envelope was a bullet. *A bullet!* And a note intimating that this would be my reward if I had the guts to play well in the Final and that if I excelled I would be 'floored by the IRA'.

We had to take the threats seriously, especially one of this kind. At the same time, I said to myself: it simply isn't possible that somebody would be crazy enough to kill a bloody football player! I mean, I admit I am a complete lunatic and I like to provoke, but in the end I'm just a lousy footballer! A simple sportsman who only wants to win a trophy. That's all.

Full of confidence I entered the arena. Felt sharp as a knife. All I wanted to do was win the bloody game, which, in the end, we did. We trashed them 5–1, with one goal scored by yours truly – a free-kick after 33 minutes, which gave Gordon Marshall no chance. From over 30 metres it went straight into the far end of the goal like a real bullet. Unlike the one the 'IRA' had in mind for me, thank God!

And that's how I dealt with the death threat, ladies and gentlemen. Maybe someone else would have run away. Not me.

The idea of letting all those magnificent Rangers fans down never crossed my mind.

And, no, I never regretted my little joke at the press conference. Because at that moment it genuinely reflected my mood. I was happy, overjoyed, to be part of the big Rangers family, and proud to follow in the footsteps of legends such as Paul Gascoigne, Graeme Souness, Ally McCoist and Brian Laudrup.

That presentation, by the way, was just for show, for the press. Sitting between David Murray and Dick Advocaat, I signed the contract. Well, a piece of paper. The real autograph had been signed three months earlier. In secret.

It was a three-year contract, which made sense. The period was long enough to see whether I would adapt to Rangers, long enough to achieve something in terms of prizes and long enough for the club to work out if I was making any progress.

Which I didn't in the beginning. The prelude to the new season had barely begun, but I already had doubts about the transfer. Three years at Glasgow Rangers: would I be good enough?

This was, literally, a completely new ball game!

With AZ, I'd always been the main man. Everything I did, I did well. Out of ten passes, at least nine and a half reached their destination. But in Glasgow? In Glasgow, all of a sudden I was crap! An amateur. A bungler. I couldn't even kick a ball to a guy who was practically standing next to me.

What had happened? I felt like a total jerk. And I was close to desperation.

What had happened, of course, was a change of skill level. After all, the gap between Glasgow Rangers and AZ is as deep as the Grand Canyon. Three years earlier, I was playing in the Dutch First Division against the likes of Telstar, Haarlem, TOP Oss and RBC, the local pride of Roosendaal. Now I was kicking balls on behalf of the mightiest club in Scotland. And to any reader who thinks the Scottish competition is a Mickey Mouse League, well, think again! You simply don't get it tougher than in the land of the brave. It's a battlefield there.

So, I was struggling – big time. Undisputed low point: the pre-season match against Livingston, which we lost 1–3. All three goals in the Almondvale Stadium were made by my direct opponent that day.

And that wasn't even a turning point! I continued to play like a sack of potatoes, in matches as well as on the training pitch, and I started to ask myself: why oh why did you come to Rangers this early in your career? Despite that magic word in the club crest, you aren't ready for it yet. Or are you? No, you aren't! Hell, you should've stayed at AZ, you moron!

On top of that I still didn't have a satellite dish, so I couldn't watch Dutch television. All my certainties had gone. I missed home.

And then, five matches into the season, there it was: my very first Old Firm game! Too early? Maybe not. After all, Dick Advocaat still believed in me. I knew I'd played crap against Saint Johnstone, Kilmarnock, Saint Mirren and Dunfermline, but Dick never let me down. Well, that's what Dicks are for, eh? Seriously though, he kept supporting me. Never failed. 'You're doing fine, Fernando. Don't despair, it's gonna be all right.'

So I was in the team on that memorable day of 27 August 2000 at Celtic Park. I knew it had to happen there and then. I knew that playing well in the only game that really matters would make life with Rangers a lot easier. All I had to do against Celtic was bring out the Fernando from previous years. I simply had to be able to play the way I did before the transfer.

Easier said than done. The night before the game, I could hardly sleep. Largely thanks to some Celtic supporters who kept sneaking into our hotel to set off the fire alarm! Every single time, we had to get out of bed and stand on the pavement in our pyjamas. Well, the last two times I thought, screw you, and stayed in bed.

Insomnia aside, that Celtic–Rangers would be a game I'd prefer to forget. I blew it – completely. After no more than twenty minutes, Dick took me off the pitch. He could see that I didn't stand a chance against Bobby Petta, Celtic's Dutch left-winger. So, instead of growing into the match I was more or less growing out of it. Not a single bit of confidence did I gain that afternoon. And when I saw my substitute, the Turk Tugay Kerimoglu, peeling off his training suit, I totally lost it.

'Why, Dick? Why the fuck are you doing this to me?'

Within eleven minutes the score was 3–0. And all of the goals had started on my side of the pitch. Credit to Bobby Petta, who did a wonderful job and provided Chris Sutton, Stiliyan Petrov and Paul Lambert with solid support.

Still, I was cursing when I noticed my number on the substitutes' board. 'Why me?' I grumbled.

No need for an answer there, really. I'd played like a damp newspaper, but there were still about 70 minutes to go. Plenty of time for me to turn the tables. Things could change, couldn't Dick see that?

No, he couldn't.

It was the biggest humiliation in my entire life. I can still hear, no, feel the whistling from the stands. To make things worse, being a right-wing defender I had to walk all the way from the far side of the field to the tunnel. It felt like a lifetime.

I got a handshake from Dick, but that didn't cheer me up one bit. On the way to the dressing room, I smashed a door to pieces. One of those beautiful old ones, pure craftsmanship – hope they still had the receipt.

I was furious at everybody. Everybody but me, predictably. It was everyone else's fault, not Fernando's. Hell no! I was Fernando Ricksen, footballer par excellence. It wasn't me who'd messed it up; it was my fellow teammates, the filthy press hounds, the supporters and, above all, Dick Advocaat, who had been stupid enough to take me off the pitch.

It was Jim Bell, our incomparable kit man, who managed to calm me down. He put me under the shower, and minutes later, along with the hot water, my anger went down the drain. But it was one very shitty day. The Hoops gave us one hell of an ear-bashing. In the end it was 6–2, and Barry Ferguson had been sent off.

The game was dubbed the 'Demolition Derby' – and it was!

On the way back, in the coach, I kept my mouth shut. For once, I knew that saying nothing might be the best thing to do.

How different things would be six months later, on 11 February 2001!

Once again I had to face Bobby Petta in yet another edition of the ongoing soap opera called the Old Firm. I hadn't forgotten our first confrontation. How could I? The Scottish press kept reminding me about the Demolition Derby. They didn't stop writing about what a complete waste of money I'd been. So I had told myself that whatever happened, I wouldn't let Petta make a fool out of me again. Once was enough!

By this time, I was a completely different player – stronger, full of confidence. So I made a plan to stop Petta. The plan consisted of two words: whack him.

So the moment he wanted to sneak past me, I hit him. Hard. It was my way of giving him a wake-up call. Didn't want to cripple the guy, no way. It was just a reminder: not today, Bobby!

I never really did have any scruples when it came to booting the odd pair of hairy legs. Ask Derek Riordan. If he still can talk, that is. Let me take you back to Thursday, 5 February 2004, and the League Cup semi-final against Hibernian, at Hampden Park. I elbowed the guy. And I did it so hard I swear I could hear his nose cracking like a bag of crisps. It looked awful, like a piece of modern art with splashes of red paint all over the canvas. Riordan was out, no doubt about it.

Well, I thought he'd asked for it. I was already past him, with the ball, but he kept pulling my shirt. And if you pull my shirt, I have to get free. And if I get free, chances are you'll connect with my elbow. By accident. Or at least that's what I always said to the ref. This time, Kenny Clark didn't even give me a yellow card. There was just red for Riordan – all over his face.

Guess what? Despite the fact that Riordan was floored, screaming like a pig at a slaughterhouse, we were allowed to continue playing. No intervention by the ref! So Shota Arveladze could play the ball to Michael Mols, who managed to score. Too bad we didn't make it to the final though. Out we went on penalties, with Frank de Boer missing the crucial one.

Still, it wasn't game over for me. Not long after the final whistle I found myself at the police station. The thing is, referee Clark hadn't seen anything unlawful, but the television viewers had . . . especially those who slept in Celtic pyjamas. Until that moment I didn't know that in Scotland you can declare a crime anonymously, which is exactly what half of Glasgow did! For them it must have been Christmas and Saint Patrick's Day all in one: not only did their beloved footballers beat their sworn enemies, they could also kick one of them in the nuts. And how eager they were to do so! Luckily the coppers just warned me to 'Never do that again, son.' And out I walked, a free man again.

Still, that wasn't the end of it, as experts from the Scottish Football Association started to analyse the footage of the clash. The outcome was that I had done it on purpose, so four weeks later I was asked to pay a £10,000 fine. And I was banned from playing the next four games.

All this for an incident that I hadn't even been reprimanded for by the referee . . . Well, not quite. The punishment had everything to do with my past.

I still had a conditional sentence from an incident in November 2000 when I had left Aberdeen's Darren Young in a bit of pain. Back then, that skirmish cost me five matches. And that was well deserved, I admit, for I don't think I've ever hurt anyone more than when I put my studs into Darren Young's flesh. Not very nice of me, I agree, but just as with Riordan it was a case of: he asked for it!

Darren was an irritating opponent. Very irritating! The Ricksen type . . . But there was one difference between us: I never tried to harm anyone on purpose. Well, until that Sunday in November, that is, in Aberdeen's Pittodrie Stadium. That's when I encountered Darren Young, a guy with an unhealthy appetite for hurting people and causing pain and misery, just for the sake of it.

This afternoon was no exception. He was bugging me non-stop, with nasty tackles from behind: both legs, and always aiming for the calves instead of the ball. I kept telling him, 'Please stop it, or you will regret it!' No reaction. Being a proper hard bastard, he continued kicking me. And after the fourth assault I had had a gutful. I told myself, He's gonna get one! Always hitting me from the back only, I thought was cowardly. Be a man and have the guts to face me, for Christ's sake!

I knew Young would go after me for round five, so I kept an extra eye on him. I also knew it would just be a matter of time before he regretted the fact that he'd tried to break my legs. So, the next time he came after me like a bloodhound, ready to bite my legs, I counter-attacked in style: with a backwards kick the world hadn't seen since the halcyon days of Bruce Lee. Bull's eye!

Okay, it had nothing to do with football as such, but it was just a matter of getting even. He'd kicked the shit out of me for God knows how long, so now it was payback time. And I did a pretty nifty job, as referee Mike McCurry didn't even give me a yellow card!

Too bad the match was shown on television . . .

So there I was, suited and booted, at the SFA headquarters. 'It was self-defence, gentlemen!' I piped up. 'Nothing but self-defence! It was him or me. He was determined to kick me out of the stadium, so I had to do something before he could achieve that!'

I could see they weren't too impressed, so I added something to my personal plea. I told them how weird it was to punish a player purely by checking television footage. 'If you do that, why not study it to see whether it was a penalty or not as well? And how about all this fake diving? It's easy to give that a second look on the telly too!'

I think they felt I had a point there, as in the end I was only suspended for two games. Case closed? Oh no! Within days I was suspended for another three matches. The reason: my comments on www.icons.com. On that website, frequented by a lot of footballers, I had written that Young was a mean bastard 'who only wants to hurt his opponents'. And somebody like that, I vented, simply needs to be kicked himself.

It was the truth, the whole truth and nothing but the truth. But the SFA weren't going to tolerate it. Hence three more games without slipping into my boots.

I was stricken by this punishment. Didn't get it at all. Here I was, facing a woman who sentenced me to three more games on the bench. A 70-year-old woman, more to the point. 'Respect?' I growled at her. 'What has this got to do with respect? How dare you punish me like this? On the strength of a comment on a website? You don't even know what a website is! You don't even know how to write the word website!'

And then I totally lost it. I went off on a tirade – about freedom of speech and how the Scottish version differs from the British one.

'Please, Fernando, behave,' whispered the Rangers officials, who were sitting next to me. I pretended not to hear them. Instead, I went on and on about the 'British banana republic' and how I had the goddamn right to write what I felt, as long as it was the truth. And this was the truth. Young was a foul player who always wanted to do you harm, so it would be *unthinkable* that I would ever apologise to him and . . .

It was a waste of time. They were not impressed. So that meant a total of five suspended games. What a shit season!

And now an edifying word to the youth. No, Uncle Fernando isn't an antisocial arsehole. Please, listen. I know I'm a tough player, but playing tough is part of the game. It has been for years. In the past – to be precise, the early seventies – there were my fellow countrymen 'Iron' Rinus Israël and Theo 'The Tank' Laseroms, who formed the heart of the Feyenoord defence. If they clashed with you, you could retrieve your bones from the terraces. And don't forget: that little fellow Dick Advocaat was a meanie too! It's just that we had about one camera per game back then – and not even all matches were captured on film! So lots of their antics remained unseen. When I hit somebody's ankle it's captured by God knows how many cameras. What they did in the past was just as bad – sometimes even worse – as what we do today. But we have the disadvantage of having everything televised. Fernando Ricksen was *not* the guy who invented the death kick, okay?

So, back to my second Old Firm game and back to the moment I floored Bobby Petta. That was not to do him any harm. Why should I? Bobby was a top guy. We even went out for a drink once in a while. Unlike Young, Petta wasn't a crook at all. Oh, Young, there we go again . . . At one point I was called 'The Meanest Footballer in Scotland'. I still don't get it; I wasn't half as irritating as that Young bloke.

Okay, back to Bobby Petta – again! Couldn't touch him too much after our little bump, as referee Hugh Dallas had given me a yellow card. So I had to play carefully for the rest of the game – and that was exactly the instruction Dick Advocaat gave me.

But 'Ricksen' and 'playing carefully' simply don't go together and shortly before half-time I gave Tom Boyd a 'little cake', as we say in the Netherlands. Well, that was it. Second slice of cheese from Mr Dallas and off I went, to a premature shower. Again. Just like six months before. With one significant difference: no handshake from Dick Advocaat this time. He didn't even look at me when I walked past him. Well, I couldn't care less. I was fuming. Not with myself, but with the big, bad world, the world that was always against poor little Fernando.

Dick, of course, was part of that world. More to the point, he was the leader of the pack, my biggest and baddest enemy at that very moment. So, as soon as he entered the dressing room at half-time I went for his throat. I literally jumped over the masseur's table to try to punch him in the face. But he didn't back off, oh no. He stood his ground and started growling at me. He was just as angry with me as I was with him. Dick did his best to stay calm and said, 'Come to my office tomorrow, so we can talk about this like grown-ups. But not now, as I have a team to coach, in quite an important match.'

I couldn't wait that long though. I wanted to confront him that very moment. Okay, I don't really think I would have punched him, but I was totally up for a verbal battle. Hence my yelling and cursing. Why, for Christ's sake, couldn't I play every week? I would be so much better if I could, so much more in shape. Why the hell did I have to sit on the bench for 90 minutes when we played the same Celtic side four days earlier, in the semi-final of the League Cup?

It was as if all my pent-up frustration had made me erupt like a volcano. After all, it had been a disappointing six months. Times were so bad that I seriously thought about quitting football. I couldn't deal with the pressure any more. I was dreaming of going back to Limburg to become a bricklayer. God, I loved the idea of a nine to five job! Do your thing in the daytime, have your dinner at six and spend the rest of the night watching telly, without millions of people looking over your shoulder. To hell with all the money I was making as a footballer! As a bricklayer I would have less cash, but less worry!

Never did it, though. I was a professional footballer and I had a contract. With Glasgow Rangers. But I played badly, very badly, and I kept being sent off. I blamed others for that, especially my coach, Dick Advocaat.

So I kept screaming and screaming at Dick, 'You don't give me any confidence at all!' Which, to be honest, wasn't true. Dick was one of the few people who were good to me. It's just that I didn't see it, because I was wearing blinkers.

It was about time to take them off.

SIX

BULL'S EYE

GERT-JAN GOUDSWAARD, RANGERS' Dutch club doctor, kept repeating it: 'Play simpler, Fernando, simpler.'

It was as if those famous words of the great Johan Cruyff were echoing in the room. 'Playing football is simple, but playing simple football is difficult.'

The words of the doctor went in one ear and out the other. Playing simple, pfff . . . No intention of doing that, doc! I wanted to show off, be the star of the team. It was stupid, as I wasn't exactly Dennis Bergkamp or Lionel Messi. Actually, I was a very, yes, simple footballer! It's just that I didn't see it at the time. Correction: I didn't want to see it.

The idea of being a labourer in the team didn't appeal to me at all. I wanted to be noticed. I wanted the audience to say, 'Wow, that Fernando Ricksen is a phenomenal player!' But, in reality, I wasn't. And that was hard for me to accept.

Playing like a prima donna, like I used to do in the old days, in the streets of my hometown, wasn't possible now. Not in Scotland. Way too tough, mate! And I wasn't the only one to find out. The legendary Frank de Boer, who arrived three years after me, was a great player. Amazing record with Ajax and Barcelona, terrific defender who always stood his ground, even in his days at Galatasaray, in Turkey, and within days he found out that Scotland is completely different. There's no such thing as an easy game here! Everybody wants to beat Celtic and Rangers, so every single time you face an opponent that team appears with 200 per cent motivation. Hence every match is bloody difficult. Most of the time, beating Celtic and/or Rangers means the entire season is a success.

Never a dull moment once the ref has blown his whistle, never a quiet moment either. It's constant kick and rush. They're after you for 90 bloody minutes. Some of them resemble woodcutters more than athletes, but they have an enormous endurance. Having an away game on the not-so-flat grounds of Inverness, Aberdeen or Dundee United isn't a pleasure at all. Add to this the all-time-low feeling I was carrying on my shoulders and it was obvious that I had to talk to someone.

Gert-Jan Goudswaard was that someone.

You see, footballers come and go. They're here today and somewhere else tomorrow. So why would you discuss the things that bother you with a teammate? He may not be there for you any more, 24 hours later. Besides, most of the time they don't care about your problems anyway. Gert-Jan seemed like someone I could trust. Someone who wanted the best for me and really meant what he said. Hence my regular visits to him.

The more I came to his office for a cup of coffee after training, the more I realised the sense of what he was trying to tell me. And from my point of view it was great to have somebody with whom I could talk about the things that concerned me – about how terrible I really felt inside. So, in the end, I decided to do what he told me.

My new pal at Rangers, Bert Konterman (five years my senior and an experienced player with Feyenoord and the Dutch national team), was in the same boat as me. The press were after him too. 'K.O. NTERMAN' they wrote, in an attempt to be funny. We talked about how badly both of us were treated, but we couldn't really help each other.

So, it was just me and Gert-Jan chatting away for hours. And it worked. Within six months I had pulled myself out of the proverbial hole. And I was playing simpler, just like the doctor ordered. I was on the way back, definitely.

I realised it on the training field too. Guys were starting to kick me again. Always a good sign! It meant that I was, well, dangerous again and had to be stopped.

I kicked back, just as hard as they did – maybe a little bit harder – but nobody cared, as they were all top guys. Only Andrei Kanchelskis, that mad hatter from Ukraine, went insane when I touched him. Idiot! Go and play billiards!

Maybe it sounds weird, but my five-match ban had a soothing effect on me. It gave me a bit of time for some much needed self-analysis. In those weeks of contemplation I started to cheer myself up, saying, 'Okay, Fernando, you've hit rock bottom. Things can't get any worse. From now on, the only way is up. So, start doing what you like most again and play football like you've always done. Have fun, just like in the old days!'

It worked. I started to grow, mentally and physically. I got stronger, on the inside and on the outside. I was getting ready again – like a true Ranger. Fernando had been reborn!

Everybody noticed the difference: the fans, my teammates and Dick. 'Welcome back,' he said, with a smile.

It felt good that he'd noticed. Even better that he rewarded me too! Against Brechin City, in the third round of the SFA Cup, I embarked on a string of matches, after which I ended the season with 37 games to my name. Just a pity that we missed the title by, er, fifteen points – to Celtic.

Spoiler alert! In the next season, my second with Rangers, we would win the SFA Cup and the League Cup, followed by the treble in 2003. So, after all, my stay with Rangers turned out to be highly successful.

Too bad it happened without the man who, in the Netherlands, is known as 'The Little General': Dick Advocaat. On 12 December 2001, shortly after a spectacular victory over Paris Saint-Germain, Dick was succeeded by Alex McLeish. I won't say he was sacked. They don't sack people at Glasgow Rangers. They're too decent for that.

Besides, Dick was still welcome at the club. Basically he had been promoted. From that moment on he was our technical director.

He hated it. Dick is the kind of guy who has to feel the grass under his toes. On top of that, he didn't see it as a promotion. In his eyes, it was a demotion. So, soon after that, The Little General packed his suitcases. It was the end of four seasons at Ibrox and the end of an era.

The departure of Dick didn't come as a complete surprise. Oh no, we were fourteen points behind you-know-who and, as you can imagine, on those occasions things get tricky at Rangers. And there were always our friends from the media to stir things up.

One morning I opened up one of those lovely tabloids and burst out laughing. It was close to Christmas so they had depicted Dick as a turkey. Quite funny, to be honest, but at the same time, when a thing like that happens you know your days are numbered. You have fewer days left than a real Christmas turkey!

Not long after that, the suits at the club had something to say to us: 'Alex is our new man.'

I didn't panic when the board informed us about the changing of the guard. I was in top shape, so I was sure I wouldn't lose my spot on the pitch.

No way!

I'd heard about McLeish and his achievements at Aberdeen. Three titles and five Scottish cups in the eighties, thanks a great deal to manager Alex Ferguson. As a player, McLeish used to be a tough one, so surely he would like me.

And I was right!

'Fernando,' he said, in our first one-to-one chat, 'you are my man.'

I'd expected him to say a thing like that, but it was still great to hear it. Trust – the best thing a footballer can get. Still, I had my doubts when all of a sudden, in January 2005, I was called to his office.

'*Fernando!*'

Oh dear, I thought. What have I done now? I was thinking and thinking and . . . *Oh nooo, not that thing in Athens!*

It was one day before our Champions League clash with

Panathinaikos and some of our board members kept saying that I wouldn't have the guts to throw our chairman John F McClelland into the hotel swimming pool.

Well, funnily enough, I did!

Little did I know that he couldn't swim. Little did I know about the phone and credit card that were still in his pocket. And little did I know that the watch he was wearing was a limited-edition Rolex worth twenty grand. (Only six of them in the whole world: five dry ones, one soaked one.)

After McClelland's involuntary dive, I'd done a *Baywatch* and saved him from drowning, and I'd apologised – sincerely even!

Nah, it couldn't be the Athens incident McLeish wanted to have a chat about. After all, it had been over a year and a half ago. And McClelland had said that, in retrospect, he thought it had been a good prank. From that moment on, the new chairman had been 'one of the lads'. The only thing he didn't appreciate was my remark that 'a twenty-grand watch should be waterproof'.

What a relief. It wasn't about Athens. It wasn't even something negative. No, McLeish had a surprise for me.

'Fernando, I want you to be my captain.'

'Can you hear the drums, Fernando?' the ABBA chicks had been singing before I was born. Now, here in Glasgow, I *did* hear those drums. Although in reality, it was my heart pounding.

'Fernando?'

This little kid from Limburg, captain of the mighty Glasgow Rangers . . .

'Would you be interested, Fernando?'

Back on my feet. This was an offer nobody could refuse . . .

'I want you to be the successor of our goalie, Stefan Klos, who's injured for the rest of the season.'

. . . but I have to stay Mr Cool, so don't yell, Fernando, don't shout yeeesss . . .

'So, what do you think about it?'

. . . just act as down-to-earth as possible . . .

'Yeah, okay, fine. I'll do the job.'

And that was it. Out I walked. McLeish must have thought I was doing it against my will. But the opposite was true. I was overjoyed.

I was the new captain of Glasgow Rangers!

Not bad for a reserve player from Roda JC, eh?

Under McLeish I would have my best period at Rangers, not least because he turned me into a midfielder. In that position I was able to leave a mark on a game, much more so than as a defender.

Not only me, but the entire Rangers gang was doing all right under McLeish. Ronald de Boer, Arthur Numan, Michael Mols, Claudio Caniggia, Stefan Klos (until his knee injury), Barry Ferguson, Mikel Arteta, Lorenzo Amoruso, Shota Arveladze and Craig Moore were having some of the best years in their respective careers. Well, you don't win the treble just like that!

I have to say, the groundwork was done for McLeish when he arrived at Ibrox, by The Little General and his aides-de-camp, Bert van Lingen and Jan Wouters. I'm sure that with Dick we would have won the treble too, no doubt about it.

After Dick's departure, Jan Wouters stayed. And I was glad he did. Terrific guy. We didn't always agree on certain things, but he certainly knew how to make me a better footballer. Despite the fact that he wasn't a big name in Scotland – although Paul Gascoigne must have remembered the way Wouters smashed his orbit to pieces in the build-up to the World Cup of 1994, forcing Gazza to perform like the Phantom of the Opera for a few months – people could sense that he must have been a hero in his day. The way he joined us in little training games was amazing. There was so much life left in the old guy!

Dick Advocaat always had a vision when he was training us. Each session was well prepared. McLeish's? Well, they were a lot McLess, excuse the cheap pun. Sometimes he let us run after the ball for the entire 90 minutes. Just kick and rush, kick and rush, over and over again. Or there was this endless – and I mean *endless* – series of headers that involved just touching the ball with your forehead.

In the beginning I thought, what the heck? This is the way to train young kids, not the way you treat adults at one of the biggest football clubs in the world. But, in fact, because the training sessions were simpler, they were a lot easier for us to understand. So, in the end, we really benefited from it.

McLeish/Wouters was a match made in heaven. After 2003's treble there was the double in 2005. Together with their loyal assistant Andy Watson, the pair created a top team with aces like Nacho Novo, Sotirios Kyrgiakos, Dado Prso, Alex Rae, Marvin Andrews, Barry Ferguson, Michael Ball and Thomas Buffel. Panic struck when Stefan Klos got badly injured, but they managed to get a very good substitute for him: Manchester City (and former PSV) goalkeeper Ronald Waterreus, who stayed on the pitch even after Klos got cured. He was just too good, our Ronald.

He was also a nutter. But there's an excuse for that: he's a goalie. And we all know they're mental. Not that I was bothered. No, I like people who stray off the beaten track once in a while – in fact, even if they do it on a regular basis. Like that other madcap, Lorenzo Amoruso. Okay, he wasn't a goalie, but he was an Italian. Need I say more? He was the kind of guy who worries whether he's got enough gel in his hair. Honest! A real dandy, who kept repeating how good he was. A pappagallo through and through!

The Scots don't like that very much. The Scots want you to act normally, do your work and shut up, but as long as he was performing well Lorenzo got away with his behaviour. And he was good, otherwise you don't get to play 150 games for a club like Glasgow Rangers. But the moment things started to go downhill, he was under fire – non-stop.

Crazy man, he was. Always complaining about the discipline, especially when Dick was in charge. But, hey, I think it's completely normal to show up exactly at the time you're told to! A £50 fine for a phone that goes off inside the stadium? No big deal, rules are rules. And if the coach says you're not allowed to wear a cap? Don't wear a cap. It's as simple as that.

I always laughed when I heard Lorenzo complaining about stuff like that. I was in stitches when Dick pulled him up in the lobby of a Norwegian hotel, during a pre-season trip to Scandinavia, because his shirt was hanging out of his trousers.

'We're on holiday, aren't we?' the Little General said, full of sarcasm.

Dick was deadly serious though. 'Put your shirt into your pants – and do it now!'

Typical Dick. Rules are rules. No: *his* rules are rules!

And Lorenzo did what he was told. Of course he did.

Meanwhile, it was my fourth year in Glasgow. And I felt great. It was easy to see why. The 2004/05 season, in which I scored fourteen times and gave numerous assists to Dado Prso, was my best one ever. Everything I did went right. I even turned free-kicks into gold. I was on top of the world.

Not that success came easy. We really had to dig deep. We literally became champions in the last minute of the last game of the season. Celtic had been ahead five points, but in their last games they completely lost it. And because of the fact that they also lost their very last confrontation (against Motherwell, with two goals from Scott McDonald in stoppage time) while we kept winning (including the last match against Hibernian, thanks to a goal by Nacho Novo), we grabbed the trophy.

It was almost better and crazier than two years earlier, when we stayed ahead of the Hoops by one lousy goal. Yes, the 2005 title was even more extreme. That's because nobody thought we would be able to do it: nobody, including the Scottish FA. They didn't even make the effort to organise a replica of the cup with us in the stadium, just in case. So when we did the unthinkable, the buggers had to fly all the way to Motherwell's Fir Park to pick up the real trophy. By helicopter! As they landed in Edinburgh somebody noticed the green ribbons were still attached to it . . . What a bunch of amateurs!

But ultimately who cares? The title was ours and being Rangers' captain, I could lift the silver proof of it. And to make things even better, I was awarded 'Best Footballer in the Premier League' by my colleagues. So every time Tina Turner's 'Simply The Best' was pumped through Ibrox – Dick had ordered the song to be played before every home game – it was, in my mind, addressed to me!

Any idea how I felt? Fernando Ricksen, best footballer in Scotland ... All of a sudden I was just as much a legend as Henrik Larsson, Paolo di Canio, Ally McCoist, Mark Hateley, Brian Laudrup, Paul Gascoigne, Chris Sutton and Barry Ferguson. I was simply the best.

Maybe it was because of my attitude. Everyone could see it was perfect. I always wanted to win. Well, I had to have some attitude, as I was lacking a bit in technique, as we discussed earlier. That's why I ran so much, and so fast. In the first ten minutes of the game, I used to sprint past my direct opponent again and again and again, until he was completely out of breath. And then I'd do it again to finish him off! It never failed.

Okay, dear friends, I have to confess something: I had to share the title 'Best Player' with John Hartson, top scorer of that other Glaswegian team. Well, good luck to him. I was happy anyway. Happy that I hadn't left the club in 2000, after six rotten months. Happy that I hadn't become a labourer. 'Best Bricklayer in Limburg'? Hmm, not quite.

To top it all off, my incredible fans honoured me with the title 'Rangers Player of the Year'. I still thank them for that.

Now, they say success turns you into a different person. And it's true, in some cases. It's hard not to let it happen. When everybody tells you how great you are, day in, day out, it's easy to start thinking: yeah, they're right, I *am* great! And then arrogance takes over.

Not with me. I always stayed a normal dude, no matter how many prizes I won. I kept doing what I had to do during training sessions too. Why not? I loved training! Mind you, most of the time I was on the field 90 minutes before the others! And I stayed there for another full hour, after training had finished, practising free-kicks, corners, the lot. At times they even had to send me away!

My attitude towards the fans didn't change either. I kept making time for them, no matter how shitty my mood was. I'd always be there for them. Everyone who wanted an autograph got his autograph. Sneaking out, like Barry Ferguson occasionally did, didn't cross my mind. I found that disrespectful. After all, it's the supporters who help to pay your salary. Especially in Glasgow, where people would rather pay for a season ticket than pay their rent. Everything rotates around football. They worship you. So why on earth would you turn your back on them?

I've always respected the mighty Scots. So the moment I was about to be crowned their number one footballer, I didn't have to think twice about what to wear to the event. It simply *had* to be a kilt! A blue one. Well, you didn't expect green, did you?

Now, I have to confess to some foul play that night. I'd been wearing jocks (no pun intended) – not because I'm prudish, but because my kilt was made of sheep's wool. Way too itchy, boys and girls! I've never worn the kilt since. Not even back home in Limburg, at Carnaval. At £2000 a go it's way too precious to face litres of flying beer.

All in all, 2005 was an unforgettable year. It was the year I made it. The year I hit the bull's eye.

So, it might have been a good idea to leave then. I had won everything and reached every goal. It was perfect, couldn't get any better. So why sign another contract with Rangers?

Because that is what I did. With twenty clubs lined up for me. I could have gone to Everton, Udinese, Atletico Madrid . . . But I decided to stay in Glasgow – where things would never be as good as they'd been in 2005. With the exception of the fans, who never let me or the club down. I still salute them. They love Glasgow Rangers. And so do I to this day. That's why I wept when I heard about the club being punished for that taxation thing in 2012. Awful!

I couldn't believe that none of the other clubs made any effort to prevent Rangers from dropping to the Third Division. They could have done something, but they didn't. After which they ended up with a diluted competition. Well done! As if Hearts and Hibernian could collect as many European points as Rangers!

Anyway, in 2018 Rangers will be back in the Champions League. At least, that's what Ally McCoist says. And he's often right . . .

Looking back, I feel privileged that I've played a few Old Firm games. A few? Twenty-five in total! Rangers–Celtic is pure mayhem, but at the same time it's one big party. And the best one of all was the one on 9 January 2005 at Celtic Park. The goal I scored that day, just after half-time, was unique. The Celts were singing 'You'll Never Walk Alone', and right at that moment there was my header, from a distance of over eleven metres. They fell silent, just like that, all 60,000 of them. Unfortunately we lost the match 2–1, thanks to goals from Chris Sutton and John Hartson, but that's a minor detail.

No football game on earth – I know I keep saying it – can beat an Old Firm clash. The tension in the stadium, the emotion, the atmosphere – unbelievable. And then there's the junk they throw at you: coins, lighters, you name it. Pure madness. I once had blood all over my face after being hit by a coin thrown by a woman who eventually ended up in court. That was about as, er, unusual as the time when an Aberdeen supporter ran on to the pitch to give me a karate kick. He wasn't very experienced though.

But, hey, Ricksen, that was why you moved to Scotland in the first place, wasn't it? I wanted to win trophies, but another reason for coming to Glasgow was to experience the emotion. And, more than anything, the emotion of the Old Firm. Ronald de Boer and Michael Mols were right: in football there's nothing more exciting than a game between Rangers and Celtic. On top of that, this clash of titans had made me stronger as a footballer. Stronger and better. Exactly what I had in mind when I changed Alkmaar for Glasgow in 2000.

Unfortunately, after a while I changed into another human being too – and not a nice one. One I would come to detest.

SEVEN

OFF TRACK

AFTER SIGNING THE CONTRACT in Scotland I immediately knew where I was going to live. It simply had to be Newton Mearns, the posh village in the hills of East Renfrewshire, a ten-minute drive from the throbbing heart of Glasgow. It wasn't just where all the Celtic and Rangers players lived, it had the best and biggest houses too. It was like driving into an American movie set. Huge houses with enormous gardens and impressive driveways. I felt like I was in *Dynasty*.

It didn't take me long to make my choice. It was love at first sight with this monumental, two-storey villa. Even the price tag of £500,000 couldn't dampen my enthusiasm. Who cared about the money? I certainly didn't. I was about to make a fortune at Rangers. The future was blue – in more ways than one!

Besides, the house had four large bedrooms. Not two, not three, four! Not that I really needed them – with Graciela's regular visits to Holland I would be the only occupant for most of the time – but it was, well, just a nice idea, four bedrooms. On top of that, the building was round the corner from my teammates Ronald de Boer and Michael Mols.

This love for my new neighbourhood wasn't mutual. They hated me, the snobbish snakes who crawled on the well-tended lawns of Newton Mearns. The guy who lived behind me, was the worst of the lot. On the night of 23 November 2002 he suddenly appeared on my doorstep – and not to invite me to a neighbourhood barbecue!

He was fuming. 'I'm gonna destroy you!' he hissed.

Welcome to Newton Mearns!

Well, he had a point, to be honest. I kinda knew why he was about to explode, here, in the middle of the night.

It must have been the fireworks. Big, flashy rockets that I'd ignited a few minutes earlier.

'You can't do this!' he growled, pointing at the sky where the remains of my premature New Year's Eve celebrations were still visible, like the steam coming out of his ears.

'You've woken up all the kids in the neighbourhood!' he yelled, thus waking up the last few who had slept through my little bit of late-night noisy naughtiness.

He didn't impress me though. C'mon guy, give me a break! Yeah, I know it's one in the morning, but, hey, it's Saturday! No school on Sunday, mate. The kids can sleep in, remember? And, besides, I'd launched the rockets from my own friggin' garden! And in my garden I make the rules!

For Christ's sake, it had been a marvellous spectacle! Hadn't he noticed? These were beautiful fireworks, not some cheap shit! Lots of neighbours had enjoyed the show. I'd heard one 'Oooh!' after the other. It was like a bunch of Chinese gunpowder merchants had come to Newton Mearns to demonstrate the latest developments in the fireworks industry. Although, in reality it was just Fernando Ricksen from the Netherlands – who loved all the nocturnal attention and was growing a few inches on this particular night.

Standing there, downing a few bottles of beer, I fully understood the appreciation most fellow Newtonians had for the show I put up. For these were real rockets. Not kids' stuff. Not with Fernando, guys! These fireworks were like the ones the Swiss use to create avalanches, in between melting cheese. And the *noise* they made! My fireworks must have woken up the Loch Ness Monster, such was the impact of the explosions. So, yes, I could understand the situation with poor old him and the children. Not that I had any remorse at the time.

When I was a kid myself, I'd never had any fascination for fireworks. Okay, I launched the occasional end-of-year party cracker, but that was about it. The biggest difference with the situation in Newton Mearns was the added liquid that was flowing through my veins. Back then it was soft drinks and milk; now it was booze. And a Fernando Ricksen on the piss gets cocky.

That night was no exception. 'Bring on the second box!' I could hear myself shouting. (The boxes were two metres square, just to give you an idea of the firepower.)

As the Dutch guys who were staying with me that weekend climbed up the stairs to get yet more ammunition, I hopped towards the fridge to get a fresh beer, already anticipating Armageddon Part 2.

My neighbour, however, didn't like the idea one bit. He kept yelling at me, in an attempt to make me stop the show.

Not a wise thing to do to me, I told him. Being aggressive to me may lead to trouble. Avoid trouble and shut up: that was what I tried to make clear.

But he didn't get the message. He kept screaming at me and, even worse, let his hands do some of the talking.

And with that he crossed the line.

'Keep your dirty hands off me!' I spat at him. In my rage I started pushing him. Pulled his shirt too. I was angry, you know. But despite shaking him like a rattle on the Ibrox terraces, he didn't back off. On the contrary. With all the weight he was carrying around he tried to prevent me from launching another squadron of missiles. When he didn't succeed he exploded – just like the rockets.

And then came the threats, which I decided not to tolerate. 'What do you want?' I yelled at him. 'What the fuck do you want?'

There was a little bout of fisticuffs too. And no real answer on his behalf. Well, whatever he wanted was irrelevant by now. All colours of the rainbow were already gathering above the roofs of good old Newton Mearns, and the noise was simply deafening.

Off he went. Good night, neighbour, no need to wake up the kids now! I was even waving at him as he left. Very, very childish, I know, but so much fun.

By that time, the beer had taken its toll. I was, I admit, completely rat-arsed. And I was still plastered when the cops arrived at about five in the morning.

Why were they there? Because of the fireworks? No way. In Scotland such a thing is anything but illegal. That's exactly what I mumbled to them, as they questioned me on my doorstep. August, June, March: there isn't one month in which you're not allowed to light a firecracker. Especially when you're on your own property.

Nevertheless, it was the rockets, they told me. More precisely, the complaints about them. So they gave me a warning: don't try this at home any more, kid.

As the officers made their way out, I took a radical decision. I decided not to open the third box of fireworks. As a wise man once said: enough is enough.

Unfortunately, this is not where the story ends, as I did get a fine. In October 2003 Paisley Sheriff Court ordered me to part with a hard-earned £7,000 after being charged with 'assault and breach of the peace'. In other words, for causing a bit of commotion and redoing my neighbour's shirt. No word about the fireworks.

Since then, they have changed the law, and now the people of Scotland are no longer allowed to set off firecrackers, other than in the period around New Year's Eve. I'm not proud of it, but it's kinda funny to think that one noisy night in my garden has changed life in Scotland for ever. They could've called it Fernando's Law, for that matter.

Enough of Newton Mearns – a bunch of filthy rich people who can't take a joke. Because that's what it was, a joke. The work of a rascal, and childish more than criminal. Anyway, I swapped the place for an apartment in the heart of Glasgow. Right across from the Scottish Exhibition and Conference Centre, on one of the banks of the mighty Clyde, I found a two-storey penthouse with a view to die for. Half a million pounds it was. I paid with a smile. No need to wrap it up, sir.

You see, I'm a city guy at heart. Always been. It's the buzz that I need. The idea of always being close to where the action is and having the city on your doorstep – literally. Pubs so close you could crawl home after last orders. And, most important of all, there was Mr Singh's Indian restaurant on Elderslie Street, owned by Bobby Singh. The curry was so good, you could eat there on a daily basis. Which is exactly what I ended up doing. No time to cook, most of the time, and no desire. So it was down to Bobby's for a nice chicken tikka. And a pint of Kingfisher.

I was so fond of Bobby's cooking that I didn't hesitate to call him when I was stretching my legs in Southern General Hospital, in September 2003. I had ended up there after an unfortunate encounter with my Norwegian teammate Henning Berg during a Champions League match against VfB Stuttgart. A collision of skulls, you might say, and not recommended, dear reader. I'd been unconscious for a few minutes, hence my transportation to the hospital. Which, obviously, isn't a restaurant. Indeed, the hospital food was so bad that I simply had to call Bobby. And within half an hour he arrived with a plastic bag full of the tastiest tandoori treats this side of the border. Needless to say the doctors and nurses were not amused. Try getting rid of the smell of a spicy chicken tikka masala in a hospital ward!

But the food wasn't the only reason for frequenting Mr Singh's. Apart from the nutrition, it was the safe environment that appealed to me. At Bobby's place I could eat and drink without being ambushed by fans or scrutinised by members of the local press. Okay, I had to sit behind a curtain, but I didn't care. It was worth it. No offence to the supporters, but a moment of giving an autograph is a moment of not eating a tikka. And as I never refuse anyone an autograph, that would mean no food for Fernando. Or at least no hot food.

After eating I often went upstairs for a game of pool. Bobby didn't have a traditional billiards table, like my granddad in Heerlen, but pool was a good alternative. I must have spent hours and hours in that room, shooting one ball after the other into a pocket. It became like my second home. Sometimes it felt more like a members' club, as the place became quite popular among footballers, both Celtic and Rangers. However, I didn't feel the need to mingle.

Apart from being my private chef, Bobby Singh became my buddy, my drinking pal, as unlike my other Glaswegian friend, Victor Morgan, Bobby liked to party. Backstreet boy Victor was much more serious than Bobby. Thanks to that, he was capable of helping me when I was in trouble. Which happened quite often, I confess. I even let him sell my house in Newton Mearns. I trusted him more than I trusted myself.

With Bobby I went on the piss, whether he wanted to or not. I sometimes had to convince him, but for some reason I always managed to talk him into it – and out of the house.

Graciela didn't like Bobby very much. According to her, he was a bad influence on me. I thought it was the biggest rubbish I'd ever heard. In my eyes Bobby was a top guy. Pure class. In Glasgow he knew everyone and their dog, and it was always heaps of fun when he was around. I liked him from the moment I met him. Lovely bloke and loyal as hell. The times he's been approached by journos to dig up some dirt about me, and he never gave them what they wanted. Paparazzi, who circled around my house like flies on shit, always got a bit suspicious when they hadn't seen me for days. On those occasions, they always called Bobby to find out what had happened to that guy Ricksen. But Bobby always said he didn't know – even when I was sitting next to him. I couldn't help laughing my head off, every time he did that. At the same time I knew: this is a proper friend, someone I can trust.

Bobby didn't even help Alex McLeish. When, in the autumn of 2003, the coach asked him to talk to me about my behaviour – more to the point, my misbehaviour – demonic laughter filled the space around them.

'Do you know how old Fernando is?' Bobby said.

'Yes,' McLeish answered. 'He's 27, almost 28.'

'Exactly,' Bobby said. And then he explained to him that a person of 27, almost 28, is an adult. 'And you don't tell an adult what to do and what not to do. That's the kind of thing you say to a child. Your own child.'

McLeish fully understood what Bobby meant, but didn't want

to give up. Yet. So he kept asking Bobby to talk to me. But Bobby kept refusing. 'It's Fernando's own responsibility,' he said over and over again. 'And apart from that, I'm not a traitor.'

And Bobby was right. There was no need to discuss my deeds. Not as long as I performed well on the pitch, which I did. Okay, I had a so-called 'flamboyant lifestyle', but none of my antics ever influenced my achievements on the pitch or the training field. Because I had this unique skill: I could drink myself silly overnight and still train like a maniac, the next morning. Even without sleep.

Actually, I gave 200 per cent during training, just to hide the fact that I'd been on the piss all night. I never let McLeish down. Never! And he knew it. Still, on more than one occasion Bobby must have thought I was a total nutcase. Like, for instance, the day I shot him.

Yes, shot him.

All right, it was only an air pistol, but still . . . those tiny little pellets hurt, you know!

Normally a vase would be the target, or a pot from the kitchen. But, see, I get bored easily, so I decided to go for livestock instead. Great fun! For me, that was; not so much for poor old Bobby. He didn't quite appreciate the fact that I shot him in the neck. He had to walk around with a red spot in his collar for weeks, poor bastard.

By the way, it was quite unusual that the two of us were at home together, that day. Normally we were painting the town red, instead of his neck! Bobby knew every single tile in Glasgow and, more important, the pubs and clubs they led to. We ended up in the weirdest places, the last one always being Seventh Heaven, a strip joint on Elmbank Crescent, around the corner from Charing Cross. It was as if we owned the place.

I could always lean on Bobby – literally! Every time I was smashed he would drag me home. Well, he had a key to my apartment anyway, so why not let him use it? Friends for life, me and Bobby, and not to forget, his charming brother Satty.

Bobby was a massive football fan. Always in the stadium, long before I arrived in Glasgow. He never asked me for a ticket though – Mr Singh had his own Skybox at Ibrox.

And not just at Ibrox . . . Believe it or not, the guy even had a Skybox at Celtic Park! Just to watch the Old Firm. Bobby wasn't too keen on the Celts, so he wouldn't be there on regular match days. When the striped ones were playing Hearts or Aberdeen, Bobby's Skybox would be filled with some of his best customers.

Wherever Rangers went, Bobby went. He even flew on the same plane as the team! And that included away games in the Champions League. Nobody objected, as everyone loved Bobby, especially my fellow countrymen Arthur Numan, Ronald Waterreus and Giovanni van Bronckhorst.

Anyway, Bobby and the Dutch got along very well. He even shook hands with Pierre van Hooijdonk, Regi Blinker, Bobby Petta and Jan Vennegoor of Hesselink who were Celtic players. They ate at Mr Singh's on a regular basis. And why not? At Singh's everyone was at ease. Just ask Sean Connery . . .

After leaving Scotland, I more or less lost contact with Bobby, which was a real shame. However, recently we got in touch again, and I was happy to find out the old bugger was still alive, especially after he told me he'd almost died after a very complicated kidney operation.

Anyway, back to my transfer from Newton Mearns to Glasgow City. That was one joyous moment for my neighbour, I guess, and Celtic's Alan Thompson probably cheered too when he saw the back of me. Nah, we never had any real problems being neighbours. I went for his throat once, during an Old Firm game, but that was only because both of us wanted to win. Call it good sportsmanship.

Once in a while – well, more than once, to be honest – Thompson missed a penalty. Like at the end of the 2002/03 season against Kilmarnock, ten minutes before the final whistle. Because he failed from the spot, Celtic missed the title. The new Scottish champs, with 95 goals to the Celts' 94, were that little old team called Rangers. Thanks, neighbour!

As I mostly lived on my own during that period, my home became a watering hole for my teammates. Not too sure what Graciela thought about that, but she wasn't around much anyway. Some players just crashed out on the spot, which wasn't a problem, as the house was huge. As a service to my beloved guests, there was always plenty of booze around. They loved it – especially the Scots.

The Dutch were a bit more – how should I say this? – reserved, which was quite understandable, as they were living there with their families. De Boer and Mols lived round the corner from me, so those two always left the party before it really started.

Mols wasn't in a party mood anyway. After bumping into German goalkeeper Oliver Kahn during a Champions League match in 1999, his knee was fucked. For Michael, it was the beginning of the end. After months and months of rehabilitation he finally got back into the squad, but during his remaining three seasons at Rangers he never became the player he was before the injury. It was very sad, as the old Michael Mols was one of the best players we had, scoring the most fantastic goals. And it wasn't just quality, it was quantity too. In his first months in Glasgow, he had a 100 per cent score rate. Amazing footballer.

Back to May 2003, and the celebrations after winning the title, or to be more precise, the celebrations after the celebrations. We didn't stop once the official part of the programme was over. Oh no, it was: hail a few taxis for an after-party chez Fernando!

So off we went to Newton Mearns, but not via the usual route.

'Please turn off here,' I told the cab driver, as soon as we entered the estate.

Eyes like saucers in the back seat. 'But, Fernando,' one of my teammates said, 'this isn't your house!'

'I know,' I grinned, 'but I think we're obliged to say thank you to a very special person.' And with those words I left the taxi and walked up to Alan Thompson's front door with my fellow Gers close behind.

I told the guys to stand in front of his window, and then I bent down and opened Thompson's letterbox. I took a deep breath and then started to shout: 'Thompson! You're a loser! You can't take a penalty kick! Loser! Loser!'

And the boys started singing – completely out of tune, as you would expect, in fact you could hardly call it singing – but it was heard all over Newton Mearns. Especially because it was one in the morning.

And Thompson? Great sportsmanship, once again. He waved at me and even had a little smile on his face. Respect! I don't think I would have reacted in the same way if a thing like that had happened to me.

Over the years I'd come to the conclusion that Scottish football humour differs from the Dutch version. Scots are a lot, well, more sensible than us cloggies. Nevertheless I decided to keep joking the way I was brought up, Dutch style. And, boy, did I do some silly things! I loved to provoke McLeish by setting off his car alarm. He'd go berserk every time he heard his vehicle bleeping. And I used to nick car keys, so that I could change the parking spot. That caused me some bellyache, I can tell you. The sight of one of my teammates desperately looking for his car was always hilarious!

Most of the time, our Spanish forward Nacho Novo, Michael Mols' successor in 2004, was the victim of my pranks. I can still see him wandering around the parking lot, hands up in the air. Priceless! But, being the good bloke I am, I always appeared after a while to tell them where I had parked their property. And, most of the time, they thought it'd been a good prank. They never did anything to my car, by the way, but every now and then I would find my boots glued to the ceiling. Well, that's football humour for you. Take it or shake it. And in team building, this kind of entertainment is the cement.

That's why I'm so glad to have come across someone like Arthur Numan. Top defender, world-class, but also a master when a laugh is much needed. Like a leech, he could 'suck the blood from under your nails', as we say in Holland, but it was always done in good spirit.

Especially when we went out for dinner, when we would see the prankster he was. As we thought it was too much hassle to split bills every bloody time, we got the idea of playing cards with our flexible friends. We'd throw our credit cards on the table, and then Arthur would mix them up and pick out one, with his eyes firmly closed.

The player whose credit card was chosen would be that evening's sugar daddy.

I've no idea how, but for some reason it often turned out to be Ronald Waterreus's plastic. And he absolutely hated it, being the stingy git that he was. You know what I mean, the type of guy that uses toilet paper on both sides and barks in his own garden to save the expense of a dog. There was only one person who had to pay more often than our curly-haired goalkeeper, and that person was me. I didn't have a clue how. Fifteen cards on the table, and eight times out of ten mine was the chosen one. It must have been some kind of magician's trick, no doubt about it, but I never found out how it happened. I never complained though, as I had plenty of cash at the time.

By the way, there was another reason why I never had to search for my car in the Rangers' car park. There simply wasn't one there, as I had lost my driving licence. It was 2003, and I was directed to the passenger's seat for twelve months, having whacked a lamppost while being intoxicated. (Well, that's what the judge said.) Okay, I did drive my Jeep into one of those iron things, and even worse, I almost parked it inside Craig Moore's living room! But I wasn't drunk that Crimbo Eve: two glasses of wine, your honour, no more. Graciela can testify.

It had simply been a case of extremely childish behaviour. It was snowing that night, like on an old-fashioned Christmas card, and I decided to see what the possibilities were with my new car on the white stuff. You know, doing the *Top Gear* thing, going from one side of the road to the other, pulling the steering wheel, pretending to be in the Paris–Dakar race . . . until the car went into a skid. I remember looking at Graciela as we did a Torvill and Dean on wheels, shortly before finding a parking spot in Moore's garden. And after the *kür* it was not us taking a bow, but the lantern.

Surprisingly enough, the car wasn't a total write-off. Neither were we. So I managed to drive home, very carefully, and poured myself and Graciela a large Bacardi. After that I went to bed with her – and the bottle.

One hour later, the doorbell rang. I had no idea who it could be. Moore? No way! He would know that I was more than willing to pay for all the damage done. Besides, I was tired, so I tried to go back to sleep. But the person on the doorstep kept ringing and ringing the doorbell. In the end, Graciela decided to take a look.

Two guys in uniform. 'Good evening, ma'am, Strathclyde Police.'

They wanted to know where I was. Graciela wanted to know why they wanted to know. They didn't want to answer that question. Instead, they started yelling at her.

Dragged from my cosy visit to Dreamland, I stormed down the stairs, only to find out that I was to be arrested. Why? Apparently I had called them 'fucking bastards'.

Policemen don't like that.

Dressed in nothing more than a T-shirt, shorts and a pair of handcuffs I was taken to the police station. Merry Christmas, Mr Ricksen!

Just half an hour after hitting the lamppost and redecorating Moore's garden with the wheels of my car, I was locked up in one of those cells I'd only seen in bad TV crime series. It even had one of those old grey shitters.

They wanted me to hand over my shoelaces. 'Why?' I asked with a smirk. 'Do you really think I'm gonna kill myself? Just let me go, guys. I'm fuckin' innocent!'

They were, unsurprisingly, not impressed. They kept me inside and woke me up every two hours for some good old questioning. As if I had just murdered someone. And, Christ, all I had drunk that night was two bloody glasses of wine! Okay, followed by six Bacardi and Cokes, but that had happened under my own roof and I'd been at home for over an hour before the cops arrived! Needless to say they refused to believe me. In their opinion, only drunks fold lampposts.

That was why I refused initially to let them breathalyse me. But, in the end, I gave in and had both my breath and blood checked. Did I feel cheated though! Not just by the policemen, but also by some members of the community otherwise known as 'neighbours', who had called the police after my Jeep kissed that lamppost. Not that it had been difficult to find out who had done it. All they had to do was follow the traces in the snow that led straight to Maison Ricksen.

So, it was a night to remember – but for all the wrong reasons. Eventually they released me, but I wasn't too impressed at being kicked out in nothing but my T-shirt and shorts, never mind the fact that it was snowing. But, hey, I shouldn't complain too much. They'd thrown me behind bars at Govan Police Station in Helen Street, which was facing my beloved Ibrox. So all I had to do was cross the street, pass the petrol station, and turn right into Edmiston Drive.

There are times in life when you don't know what to say. This particular Christmas morning wasn't one of them. I knew *exactly* what to say, as I wandered into the stadium.

'Can anybody please drive me home?'

The guard who was on duty looked as if he had seen a ghost. His mouth was so wide open I could have scored a goal in it. Thirty hours before the game against Saint Johnstone, on the morning of 25 December, one of the Rangers squad, half naked, was walking around the ground desperately looking for a ride home.

Which I got. Thanks, guys!

The game against Saint Johnstone turned out to be a great one, in which I scored my very first Rangers goal. You could say that I was, well, motivated.

Still, two and a half years later I got the aforementioned driving ban. Not that it was proven that I had been driving with six glasses of Bacardi and Coke in my stomach. The judge simply suspected it. And that's how I lost my licence for a year and had to pay a £500 fine.

Not that mine was a unique situation. Craig Moore and Barry Ferguson had been banned from driving already, and on the same day I received my marching orders, Michael Ball was sentenced to be a pedestrian too.

I'd like to explain something here: I fully understand drinking and driving is a bad combination. What if you hit a child? You could ruin so many lives if things go wrong. But, for the last time, I swear that before jumping in the car I'd only had two glasses of wine. Anyway, even my lawyer Jim Peacock couldn't help me. 'That's Scotland for you,' he said. I just had to accept the punishment.

Now the Dutch word for 'lawyer' is 'advocaat', and while Jim *couldn't* help me, Dick Advocaat *wouldn't*. He was furious, as I had breached one of the most important rules at Rangers: no drinking within 48 hours before a match.

'This has been the last time, Ricksen!' he yelled at me as I entered the stadium for the game against Saint Johnstone. 'Next time, you're out. For good!' As if this wasn't clear enough, I also received a reversed Christmas bonus of £30,000. The money went to charity, so at least one good thing came out of the whole affair. Well, that and my first goal for Rangers.

Still, I was glad Dick Advocaat was my manager. By then, anybody else would have kicked me out. Not Dick. And guess what? Since then, I have never driven with the slightest amount of alcohol inside my body. Not a single drop!

Because of the driving ban, I had to be picked up by Ronald de Boer or Michael Mols, who both lived nearby. And sometimes Bobby acted as my personal cab driver. Except for the one day I didn't arrive by car. Everyone at Rangers still talks about the special vehicle in which I showed up at the training ground that morning . . .

I think I owe you a little explanation here, don't I? Shortly before I hit that streetlight and demolished Craig Moore's garden, I had ordered a brand-new car, a BMW M3. Top stuff! There was just a little problem: because of my suspension I couldn't drive my dream car, which I had shipped from IJmuiden to Newcastle and then up to Scotland. I simply couldn't take the risk of being busted – again. So Colin McRae, the famous rally champion who happened to be my pal in those days, arranged to pick me up and take me to the club. Little did I know that he wasn't coming by car, but by, er, helicopter . . .

Needless to say I was quite excited as I jumped into his Eurocopter AS350. Shortly before take-off, I called McLeish. I told him I was in England and on my way to training. There was a sound of relief on the other end of the line. But before I hung up I wanted to know one thing: where to land?

McLeish didn't get it. 'Where to *what*? Ricksen, what the hell do you mean?'

'Well,' I replied, 'I'm coming by helicopter, you see.'

'*Helicopter?* Are you out of your mind?'

No, I wasn't. I was totally sane. Well, Colin was, more to the point. And because McLeish couldn't provide us with a decent answer, Colin decided to simply descend onto the training pitch.

I told McLeish what we planned to do.

He went mental. 'Don't even *think* . . .'

The longer the phone call lasted, the angrier he got. But my only concern was to be on time for training. I didn't want to risk a fine!

Fast-forward half an hour. I saw Murray Park below me, getting bigger and bigger. As did the eyes of the youngsters who were on the pitch. There was no real alternative, so we simply had to do it there and then.

I jumped out and ran from the youth players' pitch to the one where my teammates were about to start practising. I'd made it!

The players loved it. McLeish, however, was not that amused. He fined me on the spot.

But it was an emergency, boss!

Later, after my driving licence had been returned, I started to do some flying myself. Not in a helicopter, but in a bright red Ferrari 550 Maranello, which Colin had sold to me for two grand. Beautiful car, I was so damn proud of it. So you can imagine how I reacted after the phone call in which Graciela told me she had transformed it into an accordion. Total write-off, just outside the lovely Spanish city of Valencia. Luckily I still had my BMW M3.

Colin, on the other hand, was less fortunate. On 15 September 2007 his helicopter crashed in Lanark, just two kilometres from his home in South Lanarkshire. It was a tragic accident, in which he, his friend Graeme Duncan, his five-year-old son Johnny and the six-year-old Ben Porcelli, a pal of Johnny's, lost their lives. I was heartbroken when I heard the news.

EIGHT

GIRLS, GIRLS, GIRLS

BECAUSE I FELT INCREASINGLY lonely I began to drink more and more. Sometimes, as a new day dawned, I went straight from the boozer to the training ground. I never knew whether McLeish suspected anything or not.

In my defence: contrary to popular belief I wasn't plastered all day. And I didn't wake up with a bottle of vodka in my mouth. C'mon, you couldn't survive a lifestyle like that, especially not at a club like Glasgow Rangers. So, no, I wasn't George Best the Second or The New Paul Gascoigne. Unlike them, I could resist temptation. Sometimes – honestly! – I didn't drink for days. Most of the time I wasn't intoxicated at all, dear reader, but when I did drink, for instance after a match, I drank until I fell over. I was unstoppable, and would down anything – beer, wine, spirits – as long as it contained alcohol.

I have to set the record straight here. I did feel lonely, but I seldom went out for a drink on my own. Now, *that* would have been sad. I was always joined by some drinking buddies from the club, and it sometimes happened that we didn't have a match or training on a Wednesday. If that was the case, we went to London for a drink.

Yes, London!

Joined by the usual suspects – Barry Ferguson, Craig Moore,

Jean-Alain Boumsong – I'd fly down to the capital for two nights of adult fun. Who cared about Thursday's training? There would always be an early flight back that day, so we wouldn't miss a minute of the activities at Murray Park. Call us insane, because that is what we were. But I loved every single minute of it. I simply needed a bit of thrill seeking, and there's no better place for that than London!

It may not come as a surprise that we didn't go to London to visit Buckingham Palace or watch the Changing of the Guard. After all, we weren't bloody tourists. We were pissheads. We wanted to drink – as much as possible and as fast as possible. And being the superstars we thought we were, we didn't end up in your average local watering hole. No, it had to be Tiger Tiger or Chinawhite, the trendiest nightclubs in Soho, where at some stage we would be joined by some French *footballeurs*, friends and countrymen of Boumsong. Or so I was told. By the time they arrived, I was mostly too plastered to notice.

I was busy doing other things. You see, being a footballer at a major British club, means women find you, let's say, interesting. The moment they clap eyes on you, they want to score.

And I always let them score. I'm not that difficult. It must have been nice for them to get lucky. Lucky, in this case, meaning finding out I wasn't too smashed to perform.

Still, not every chick would go for us in London. This was, after all, the Champions League of gold digging, so a lot of them were only interested in players from Chelsea and Arsenal. Glasgow Rangers may have been a bit substandard for them.

Not so in Glasgow, where Celtic and Rangers were top of the league when it came to female attention. And it would have been very impolite to neglect that attention, wouldn't it?

So, every time a girl came up to me asking me for a ride, we had that ride – sometimes even in a car! Or we played hotel inspectors and went out to test beds. I made sure I never checked in using my own name – didn't fancy the idea of reading a review in the tabloids a few days later – and I always, always dumped my passport, jewellery and money in the hotel safe first.

Those were the encounters on neutral turf. But at times I had a home game. Yes, in my own house. Totally shameless, I know. Those legs – no pun intended! – were alternated with away games. And on one occasion, the phrase 'away game' sums it up perfectly!

It was after beating FC Copenhagen, on 27 August 2003. We had qualified for the Champions League, so there was a reason to hit the bottle. It was party time!

I got so intoxicated on tequila that night I even forgot where I lived. So when this bird suggested spending the night at her place, it seemed like the most logical thing to do.

'Hi, darling,' I heard several hours later.

I turned over and got the shock of my life.

Not because she was ugly – she wasn't at all. Call me Mr Arrogance if you want but I never pulled an ugly chick. No, it was the décor. More to the point: its colour.

Pink. Everywhere. The doors, the ceiling, the walls: literally everything had been painted pink. It was too sweet to handle! I lost it. I knew this time I'd really lost it. Where was I? I had to go! Now!

'Maybe it's better if you call a friend,' my pink lady said, as she started to make coffee.

'Why?' I replied.

'Cause you can't get a cab over here, honey. It's impossible.'

Now I was getting desperate. 'No taxi?' I said. 'Where the hell am I?'

She pointed at the window. 'Just open the curtains.'

Still glowing after a night of hot and passionate sex and wearing nothing but my Y-fronts, I opened the pink curtains – only to get the second shock of a lifetime. I expected anything and everything, but not this view! Because there, right in front of me, in all its green and white glory, was . . . Celtic Park!

Hours earlier I had picked up this girl, and for the best part of the night we'd been screwing the living daylights out of each other. And all the time this Glasgow Rangers player didn't have the slightest idea that he was having a carnal carnival on the doorstep of his biggest rival's ground . . .

I immediately closed the curtains, scared shitless that somebody would spot me.

'Maybe you're right,' I mumbled.

'And I'm Celtic too,' she said, offering me a hot beverage. 'Just like my brothers.'

I started to sweat. Not for the first time in that room, but this time it felt a lot colder.

'But don't you worry, cutie,' she whispered. 'I won't do you any harm.' And she kissed me on the mouth.

My brain went into overdrive. What to do now? Going outside and waiting for a taxi wasn't an option. The Celtic mob would lynch me. That was why I didn't know where I was. I'd never made the mistake of entering Celtic territory before, so when last night's girl directed the taxi with the two of us to her house, I didn't have the slightest idea where we were. I simply didn't recognise the area.

Well done, Rangers guy, I said to myself. You're trapped in the heart of Celtic Land!

The only guy I could think of to pick me up was streetwise Victor Morgan. And, yes, he came, within thirty minutes. As soon as I knew he was downstairs, with the motor running, I ran out of the apartment straight into his car.

'*Outta here!*' I yelled.

Victor roared with laughter. But he did manage to get me out of there without anybody noticing.

Five months later, it was Celtic away. As the players' coach turned up at the stadium, I saw the apartment and immediately remembered what had happened there. I pointed at the pink curtains and told a few teammates about my adventure. From that moment on they knew it, that Ricksen guy is totally mental!

All in all, it had been a close call. And I was still married to Graciela . . .

Bedding a bird was a tricky thing to do anyway. Some tabloids even pay women to do it for them, after which they get all the juicy details first-hand. So, every famous footballer becomes a target, especially if he's married. Like I was.

Too bad for them that I always sensed the proximity of these well-perfumed decoy ducks. They always seemed to be desperate, despite the fact that they were drop-dead gorgeous. Too obvious, girls!

Unfortunately, I didn't manage to stay out of the tabloids all the time. But then, it was almost impossible not to be spotted with a delicious blonde or brunette. You didn't even have to have sex with them – a simple photo of the two of you could be enough 'evidence'. Sometimes those women pretended to be Rangers fans. 'Please, Fernando, can I have my pic taken with you?' And an hour later the photo would be at a newspaper's desk, where reporters would knit a sensational story around it. 'One onlooker said . . .' were the main words of choice. It was always 'a friend of a friend' who provided the quotes (the fake quotes, of course). But because all the nasty bits were between quotation marks, I could never sue the filthy press hounds.

It drove me nuts. For it wasn't just once that they saw me with 'a new girlfriend', I was dubbed a 'love rat' hundreds of times! And what could I do to defend myself? Go into hiding? Now *that* would have been suspicious. Refuse every single request for a photo? Disrespectful to the real supporters. For reasons of 'safety' the papers were never obliged to name their 'source', so there was absolutely nothing I could do.

What I did do though was stop any kind of cooperation with those scumbags. No interviews any more – screw you! And they only had themselves to blame.

Each and every day I expected something in the papers, and, boy, did I get it one lovely day in spring 2002! I opened the paper and there she was: a girl with a familiar face. No doubt about it: she was the one I'd slept with just a few days earlier, in my own home. It was a wild tale of our adventures on and off the bed, raunchy stuff – hotter and steamier than the coffee the paper came with. And to prove she'd really stayed in my bedroom she described exactly what it looked like. No detail was spared. I couldn't believe my eyes. An article this big about two grown-ups having sex? Was this really news?

I admit, it wasn't a total lie. It's true that I'd picked her up in Tiger Tiger near Royal Exchange Square in Glasgow, where me and the boys frequented the VIP area, but in all honesty, we didn't have sex. Stop laughing – it's the truth! She was too drunk! I'd brought her home, without having had intercourse.

Maurice Ross and Robert Malcolm would testify for me, as this time I was not going to take it. Here was a bunch of lies that I had to refute. And with success: the tabloid had to apologise. Which they did . . . on page two, hidden away in a little corner, unnoticed by the masses.

In a way I could understand those girls. Had I been in their shoes – don't even try to imagine what that looks like! – I might have done the same. In fact, I probably would have. After all, it's an easy way to make a thousand quid, and that's a monthly salary to a lot of people.

Still, I shouldn't complain, I said to myself. This was one story of a girl who pretended you'd made the world's oldest move on her. Okay, it was a bit inconvenient, but what about the 100 times you *did* shag a strange bird and it did not make the papers? Call yourself lucky, guy.

Yes, there have been truckloads of them. Girls, girls, girls. Everywhere – and always available, because I was young, rich and famous. They wanted me, and I couldn't resist the temptation. Would you?

Still, I had one strict rule: never without a condom. Oh no, the idea of putting a bun into a British oven – 'Girl Pregnant By Rich Football Player' – well, I think you get the picture. And, man, it's tricky at times. There are girls out there for whom pregnancy is the ultimate goal. Girls who want the child of a wealthy football player and not one of some bus driver. It's nasty, I know, but it happens. Hence my ever-present packet of johnnies.

So, hands up, I was a love rat. I'm not trying to justify myself – that would be hypocritical – but I wasn't the only one. Most footballers are. And you can't blame them, in my opinion. The most gorgeous women want to meet you, and how on earth can you resist? You'd be stupid if you did! Speaking for myself, I took advantage of the situation over and over again, because of the thrill, but also because, in my opinion, you shouldn't eat the same dish every day. Back home I had the juiciest, most tender steak I could get. It's just that sometimes you feel like having a pizza – or a kebab.

I hereby officially declare that 90 per cent of the footballers I knew had sex with women they were not married to or otherwise engaged to. The one exception was Mark van Bommel. Loyal as a Labrador. Full-on, dedicated family guy. But the rest? Hey, ever asked yourself why footballers always have two or three phones? Not because they collect the bloody things!

I had two. Two mobiles. One for daily use, with a number known to Graciela, my friends and my family, and another one, er, that didn't really exist. That was the one stored under the driver's seat of my car, or in my locker at Rangers – the one that Graciela couldn't see, as it was loaded with girls' names and numbers, girls I could always call in case of an 'emergency'.

In order to collect those numbers, I only had to be me, the footballer. I swear to God I found them behind the wipers of my Jeep or Ferrari – or tucked in my trouser pocket – just like that! It happened all the time. At a press conference, the opening of a shop, a photo shoot, everywhere and anywhere! Those were the moments that I thought, my God, it's better being a footballer than a bricklayer!

It was so easy, sooo easy . . . It really surprised me at times. Like one night in 2004. Once again I was out with the boys and once again we were at Tiger Tiger. We were having a ball. And, believe it or not, after a few hours of drinking and laughing, we staggered out of the club *without* any female company. You see, sometimes it's good to have just a boys' night out. There's no need for sexy chicks all the time . . .

That feeling lasted until we reached the taxi stand. There and then, we all of a sudden decided that we could do with a girl or two. So off I shuffled towards a few. No idea who they were. Never seen them before. I simply pointed my finger at them.

'You, you and you! You're coming with us!'

As my teammates were doing the same, within minutes we had a harem of twelve gorgeous chicks. That's what fame does for you.

The destination? Well, as Graciela was in Holland, it had to be my place. Plenty of room to play. I just didn't want anybody to sneak into my private bedroom on the second floor, that was all. As I was the proud owner of a brand new bath, next to the bed, I was very careful. I didn't want anything to happen to it. In a few days' time Graciela would return and if by then the bath was damaged, so would I be.

Apart from this restriction, we were having great adult fun with those bare-naked ladies, who were performing acts on us that you normally only see in porn movies. It felt like heaven with those. . .

Wait a minute. One. Two. Three. Four. Five. Six. Seven. Eight. Nine. Ten.

Ten?

Didn't we pick up twelve of them?

Oh my God!

I immediately crawled towards one of my teammates. 'We've lost two!'

He didn't know what I was talking about.

'Look! Come count with me. One, two, three, four, five, six, seven, eight, nine, ten! We're two girls down!'

After searching the corridor, the kitchen, the loo, all over the place, we still couldn't find them.

Total panic. Until someone said, 'Your bedroom!'

And, yes, despite the fact that I'd closed the door to the holy place, there they were.

In my new bath. Both of them, giggling.

I couldn't get too angry. Actually it made me laugh. Maybe it was nerves.

Now, over the years I'd seen a lot – and I mean a lot! – when it came to women and sex, but what happened on this particular night, in my own penthouse overlooking the Clyde, was un-be-liev-able! Naked bodies all over the place. Wherever I looked I saw teammates shagging one – or two – of the twelve chicks we'd picked up near the taxi stand. In the hall, in the living room, in the kitchen: everywhere people were playing hide the sausage. Threesomes galore! It was one big orgy!

One teammate told me that it was the horniest thing he'd ever experienced. 'This is a once-in-a-lifetime,' he said. I had to agree with him. It was pure madness.

Nevertheless, I was shocked next morning when I saw the mess we'd made. Empty bottles and clothes everywhere – a G-string in my plants!

Immediately I thought about Graciela. Not that I felt guilty. It was just, well, I didn't want her to know – and that meant I had to clean the place before she came back.

I succeeded – or so I thought. The very moment she entered the apartment, a few days later, her attention was drawn towards the white wall in the corridor.

'What's that?' She pointed at a large brown stain, somewhere around knee height. It looked like a piece of modern art, but obviously it wasn't. However, I didn't have a clue how it came to be there. I really didn't. Graciela didn't believe me, which was a pity, because this time I honestly wasn't lying!

And then, all of a sudden, I remembered my Portuguese pal, who had been standing there for what seemed like hours . . .

The next morning, just before training, I asked him what the hell he had been doing in my corridor. Because of that mysterious, big brown stain. He started laughing. Then he told me how he had bonked a girl in that particular spot and how, while doing that, he had pressed her face against the wall. Off came her spray-tan make-up, thus leaving the aforementioned piece of art on my once virginal white wall.

I was in stitches.

Graciela, who must have suspected where the stain had come from, never spoke about it. Thank Christ, 'cause I wouldn't have known what to tell her! To me, however, that brown splodge was a nice souvenir from an unforgettable night.

So, yes, it's official: British birds on a night out are an extremely easy prey. They simply want to be caught by any successful, loaded hunter. Yet, those short-skirted, high-heeled bimbos are not the easiest of the lot. The most ready and willing women, believe it or not, are lawyers. I've bumped into quite a few of them at charity events and, I can tell you, those well-educated beauties in their nine to five office suits have only one thing on their mind: sex!

They crave it – and they want it fast. More than once I've been grabbed by the balls and pulled into the toilets by one of those bespectacled hotties. Added bonus: most of them are happily married, so no fear of revelation. All they ever want is their daily shot of sex and sensation. And most of the time they are one-offs, so they don't even bother giving you their phone number! Well, that was fine by me.

The numbers I did have were for the times Graciela was in the Netherlands. On those occasions I got bored quite easily, so a phone bursting with girls' names came in handy. And, you know, sometimes I just wanted to have some company over dinner. Sometimes.

Anyway, I did change my number on an almost monthly basis. Didn't want them to bother me too much. Oh, and I never, ever sent any sleazy text messages. Way too risky – they could end up in the tabloids within hours.

I never had any regrets about cheating on my wife. I simply shouldn't have married Graciela. Not because of her, please don't get me wrong! When we tied the knot on 29 September 2000, at the Eastwood Register Office in Renfrewshire, I really, really loved her. I just wasn't ready for life as a married man. I was too young and too restless. Despite the kiss that sealed our marriage, I wanted to rock and roll all night and party every day. And, above all, I wanted other women's attention.

I couldn't live a life without partying. So I couldn't have felt any better than when in 2003, after winning the treble, we partied for seven days and nights in a row. Together with the frenzied fans we drank and danced in the pubs on Paisley Road until we collapsed. And when that happened I was dragged to a bed nearby. Or maybe far away. I've no idea where exactly. I just remember that in that particular week I didn't see my house at all. We were champions, and it had to be celebrated Fernando-style with the two Bs: booze and birds. It was my life and I wanted to live it the way I did.

Yes, I was a full-blown egomaniac, and in my never-ending search for lust, by autumn 2003 I would hit the jackpot.

NINE

JACKPOT

LET'S RECAP: THE MAIN reason to swap Alkmaar for Glasgow was to win prizes. Big prizes.

I think I did quite well when it comes to that. Two titles, two Scottish FA Cups, three Scottish League Cups. And on top of that I was voted Footballer of the Year. Once again, not bad.

It's just that I wanted to conquer Europe with the Gers. I played quite a few Champions League matches – around 30 in total – but reaching the final would have topped it off. Well, at least I can say I've faced Manchester United. Now that was a memorable clash!

By that time, I was an experienced international footballer. I'd played against the likes of Internazionale, FC Porto, CSKA Moscow and VfB Stuttgart. Still, the Red Devils were in another league – a totally different ballgame. All of a sudden I found myself on the same piece of grass as Ryan Giggs, Paul Scholes, Roy Keane, Rio Ferdinand and Ruud van Nistelrooy. We lost, albeit just 0–1, but it was a magnificent experience. The atmosphere at our place was incredible that night. And I wasn't doing too bad myself either. Didn't screw it up at all. It wasn't the easiest of games, especially after Phil Neville opened the scoring in the fifth minute, but I had a pretty good evening. Giggsy was my man for the night and he didn't have a chance against me. He must have hated me at certain moments, as I didn't leave him alone for one second. Well, that's the way to do it with big stars. Don't be overwhelmed by their status, just don't let them touch the ball. It's as simple as that.

Two weeks later, at Old Trafford, we were beaten 3–0, with two goals from Ruud van Nistelrooy. I wasn't there that night – probably to the delight of that curly-haired boy from Wales!

Still, Giggs isn't the best player I've ever had the pleasure to deal with. On 5 August 2003 we had a friendly against Arsenal, at Ibrox, and on that occasion I had to face Patrick Vieira. It turned out to be the most difficult evening in my career. I mean, this guy was in-cre-di-ble . . . So good, so fast, so strong. Hardly managed to take the ball off him. And the very few times I did, he had it back within the wink of an eye. I still dream about it, I can tell you!

We lost the game, 0–3, and from that moment on it dawned on me that in order to achieve international success we had to be focused 100 per cent, each and every second. There was no time for amateurism any more. No muddling like on that fateful night in Istanbul, August 2001, when we played Fenerbahçe. It was a Champions League duel which we lost 2–1, thanks to – sorry to say it! – two enormous blunders from Amoruso. He faced Haim Revivo and Serhat Akin with the attitude of a Sunday-morning park player. Both guys could simply walk past him and score.

I was going out of my mind with rage. And I gave him a personal review of his lousy performance. He didn't want any of it, so we ended up having an argument, hotter than the spiciest shish kebab.

There had already been a bit of tension between us at half-time, as Lorenzo was blaming everybody but himself. It made me stand up and walk towards him. 'What the hell are you talking about? Just use your head, that thing where that big mouth of yours is situated, to get rid of the ball! I'll clear things after that. Just give me a nice header or two, understand? Get the ball outta there!'

He didn't. The Italian prima donna simply dived under the ball, thereby giving his direct opponent a free journey ticket towards our goal. This, and this alone, was the reason I attacked him afterwards like a raging bull. I was sick of his attitude. It wasn't personal – I was one of the few players who got along with him quite well – it was just about the lack of fighting spirit he had shown. You are a professional, for God's sake, don't act like an amateur! You can't do that to all those people who buy tickets to see you perform, people who don't earn a tenth of what you get, so roll up those sleeves and go for it!

A day later, at Murray Park, we shook hands. That's also part of being a professional.

I hate to lose. The fans noticed that – that's probably why they loved me so much and looked upon me as their favourite Ranger for a while. I never gave up. I was always ready to battle. If others didn't want to share that attitude I got angry. And in a situation like that, bad things can happen. Like when we played Paris Saint-Germain in the UEFA Cup, three months after Fenerbahçe. At one stage I got so frustrated I decked Gabriel Heinze, the Argentinian, with my elbow. Second yellow card, so off to the tie and jacket ten minutes before full-time. Stupid, I know. Let's call it the burden of a Fighting Spirit.

Rewind. Back to that evening in Istanbul. You may think I can only kick opponents, but it isn't true. I can kick a ball too. And that night against Fenerbahçe I even kicked it between the goal posts. Okay, it wasn't enough for victory, but at least with that goal I would be in the Champions League history book forever.

Still, I know I am more famous for the times that I scored off the pitch. And that reached its climax when I laid my hands – and more! – on the biggest prize I'd ever won. The jackpot.

It was Saturday morning, 11 October 2003, when I turned up at Murray Park. As I stepped out of my car I could see them already, my fellow teammates, all standing next to each other in a row, as if they were expecting the Queen. I turned around but couldn't see Elizabeth, nor Philip. It was just me. Hey, were they about to salute me?

The moment I entered the hall, the boys started to applaud. They were cheering too, and yelling. The next thing I saw was the front page of the papers they were waving. Papers with me on the front page. And although the publication had nothing to do with football, my buddies were as proud as hell. Even Alex McLeish took a bow. 'No idea how you did it,' he said, 'but this is an absolute brilliant result. I truly salute you!'

Nevertheless, the club did fine me, as McLeish had previously warned me to stay away from the front pages. The total bill for this bit of unintended media exposure was £25,000, which I had to pay almost on the spot. 'Sorry, pal,' McLeish said, 'but these are the rules.' After which he added, 'But in itself you achieved the near impossible. So well done, mate!' And he shook my hand, as if I had just been rewarded with a cup of some sort.

Well, in fact I had won a cup. A huge one. This time, pun intended!

A day earlier, I didn't know who she was. Mind you, thanks to my satellite dish I only watched Dutch television – and she was never on it. British papers, well, you know the story . . . So I had never seen her, er, face before.

I must have been the only person in the whole of Great Britain.

Katie Price, better known as Jordan, was a big shot. Still is. A glamour model with giant bazookas, well, you know who she is. Model, presenter, singer, actress, fashion designer and writer even, she was highly successful in every single discipline and therefore – I have to use the word, sorry – totally loaded. Hats off to her, especially because she can't sing, or write, or act! Katie and her hot pink Jeep were as much a part of daily British life as tea with milk. She was a woman who never failed to make headlines. The moment she wants some media attention she simply steps out of a cab without wearing any knickers. There'll always be a photographer waiting to catch a glimpse of her tattooed vagina.

As you read this – I'm guessing, as things move fast in her life! – she's happily married to Kieran Hayler, an English stripper, with whom she has a child. It's Katie's third marriage, after being the wife of Australian singer Peter Andre and English cage fighter Alex Reid. Earlier on, she'd been in relationships with my dear colleagues Teddy Sheringham and Dwight Yorke, with whom she has a son. No, never a dull moment with Katie!

So we're talking A-list celeb here – although I didn't have a clue on that beautiful Friday evening in October 2003. Just like the Rangers squad she had been invited to the Hottest Night of the Year charity event, organised by curry tycoon Charan Gill. McLeish had taken us aside for a little speech. 'Listen,' he said, 'I'm only going to say this once. Behave – every single one of you! He who doesn't will get fined – enormously!'

The crowd started grinning like adolescents going on a school trip. It was obvious that they were looking forward to the event at the Scottish Exhibition Conference Centre, where Katie Price had the honourable task of cutting a ribbon. The guys were like dogs, wiggling their tails in anticipation. They were about to see Katie Price in the flesh! Jordan, the ultimate Page Three Girl!

I didn't pay much attention to McLeish's warning. As I said, I didn't know the woman. So I wasn't going after her either. And to top it off I had the intention of not sipping a single drop of alcohol that night. So McLeish wouldn't have to worry about Ricksen making a fool out of himself – not this time.

I wasn't exactly in a party mood, to tell you the truth. Hours earlier I had received a £7,000 fine for the fireworks incident in Newton Mearns, so I was a bit fed up with everything and everybody. It was just that I didn't want to let Bobby Singh down. He was more or less involved in the organisation of the evening, so in order not to disappoint him I decided to go. 'Just a few glasses of Coke and I'm off,' I said to everybody. 'Gonna watch telly at home.'

'Don't be ridiculous,' the others said. 'You're gonna miss out on a top evening.'

However, as they say, nothing ever goes the way it's planned. There I was, sitting at a table, knife in one hand, fork in the other, ready to munch on a portion of my beloved chicken tikka, as I felt a pat on my right shoulder. I looked behind me and stared into this beautiful pair of eyes, each one made even prettier with the aid of an enormous amount of eyeliner. I saw a pair of huge boobs too. And hair, long blonde hair, with extensions, like so many British girls sport.

Okay, yes, er, I sort of recognised her. This was the girl who, earlier on, had opened the event for which she scooped the sum of £2,000. Yes, this was Katie Price, aka Jordan, the same babe I'd played 'hard to get' with, when she came up to me (for what could have been a snog) about 90 minutes ago in the VIP room. I didn't know her then, and I wanted to keep it that way. Let's not get into trouble, I'd told myself.

But, hell, that must have been what triggered her! Finally, a man who wasn't after her. On the contrary! That must have made me an interesting prey.

So, there she was, all of a sudden, behind me and my beloved chicken tikka.

'Can I join you this time? Or?'

I looked around, poker-faced. 'There doesn't seem to be a spare seat, baby,' I said, cooler than the ice cubes in my Coke. 'So that's gonna be a bit of a problem.'

'Oh no,' she sort of groaned.

The next moment I saw Jordan's perfectly shaped leg flying through the air and before I could say 'chicken tikka' she was sitting on my lap. Facing me, cowgirl-style. The UK's most wanted woman.

The white mini-skirt, the tight leather belt, the e-nor-mous jugs . . . Yes, my teammates had been right. She was simply delicious – *hors catégorie.*

I saw someone watching us from the corner of my eye. McLeish. He was moving his index finger from side to side, and I could see his lips moving. *Don't! Do! It!*

Sorry, coach, trapped! I stuck out my arms and waved, like a person who is drowning, but thank God nobody came to save me.

More and more teammates were joining our table. They sensed history was in the making here. At the same time, it was an enormous opportunity to see Jordan close up. The entire evening she had been sending drooling men away. But here she was, at my table, on my lap, on her own initiative, so it was unlikely she'd do the same now. Besides, why should she? She was having a ball! And so was I. In fact, it was so pleasant that I thought, I'm staying! And out went the Coke.

'Waitress! A pint of lager, please! Oh, and another one!'

Within half an hour I'd downed about a gallon of the yellow stuff.

Jordan didn't exactly act like a nun herself, as she deep-throated one alcoholic beverage after the other. And then, all of a sudden, she spoke those immortal words. 'Why don't we just leave the place? Just you and me on our own?'

It was more an invitation than an actual statement. However . . .

'I can't,' I told Jordan, who by now was galloping on my lap. 'If my trainer sees the two of us leaving together, he'll explode.'

'So,' she whispered, looking me straight into the eyes, 'in that case we leave the place separately and we'll meet somewhere else later on.'

'Yeah, fine,' I mumbled, my head now spinning from the amount of beer I'd had. Consequences? What consequences? I told her we could meet at a nightclub. She didn't like the idea. Not enough privacy.

'How about a lap-dancing bar? Do you know any good ones?'

Yes, you read it. Katie Price wanted to take me to a strip joint!

Needless to say, I knew a few – if not all of them. I more or less lived in the bloody places! My suggestion was Seventh Heaven, a place covered in Bobby's footsteps and mine.

'Okay,' she said. 'Meet you there.'

But we didn't. Because all of a sudden she had a much better idea: her own four-wheel drive, a Land Rover parked very discreetly at the back of the venue.

'Just jump into it. Nobody will notice. Not even your coach.'

So there I was, swaggering towards the toilet to get rid of a fair amount of the beer – at least that's what I wanted everybody to think – but in reality I was sneaking out to Jordan's car. A few seconds later we were speeding away *A-Team* style.

I was thrilled, to put it mildly. It was not the first time that I'd run away with a girl, oh no, but this was . . . different. Of course it was different. I was with Katie friggin' Price!

As we drove through the Glaswegian night I had another good look at her. What! A! Top! Bird!

Funny too, and friendly. No, I'm not bullshitting here, she really is! Not at all the bitch that you might think she is. She's just built this wall around her, because everybody and his dog wants something from her. It's self-protection. Cristiano Ronaldo and David Beckham have done exactly the same.

Later in life I asked myself the question why it had been me, of all people, she'd patted on the shoulder that night. After all, the place had been packed with good-looking blokes! I concluded it was my good manners. No, don't laugh! It's a well-known fact that some Scottish men are not exactly gentlemanlike towards women. They hardly pay compliments, even though they're free. Most of the time the members of the Tartan Army are, well, a bit impolite.

I am different.

Anyway, on a night out, believe me, Jordan is the best company a man can have. However, a relationship with this woman is something completely different. I don't think I could handle it. Not that that was the purpose of our being together. That was impossible anyway, as I was still married to Graciela: Graciela, who was in the Netherlands that night and would come back, oh God, the following day.

Not that I was thinking a lot about my marital status that night. Especially not when the two of us sat down on a comfortable sofa at Seventh Heaven, which was a very appropriate name at the time. We kissed as if it was our last day on earth.

Then, all of a sudden, Jordan had an idea. 'Let's go to the back.' No objection from me! 'But not just the two of us.' And before I could produce a question mark she waved at two Hungarian girls who, just a few minutes earlier, had been hanging upside down on a pole.

The two dancers followed us immediately.

Now, there are times in life when you wish you could freeze time – a perfect moment that should last for ever and ever. This was such a moment.

The four of us walked into a private room. The Hungarian chicks dropped their sexy, blood-red lingerie and grabbed Jordan, who was butt-naked already. The girls started kissing each other. And I was . . . well, in Seventh Heaven, as I already said.

The three naked girls put on a show for me that was beyond imagination. And all of the time I was expecting some bloke to jump in from behind the curtains screaming, 'You've been punk'd!' As it *had* to be a prank with a candid camera! This couldn't be reality.

Or was it? It was.

The chicks kept kissing and licking each other, and not a single nosy parker appeared to spoil it for me. Maybe that was because they all seemed to have an appointment the morning after, right in front of the posh Moat House Hotel on the Clyde, where Jordan was staying. And where I had to do the walk of shame, in front of ten, twenty, thirty or even more hungry photographers.

As I walked out of the hotel, unshaven and with my shirt hanging out of my trousers, I did my best to keep my cool. But it was useless. The flashlights came from everywhere – it was like fireworks on New Year's Eve. At a certain point, I couldn't see anything at all any more, as a tsunami of artificial light was thrown upon me.

So this is how Brad Pitt must feel, I thought to myself.

The next moment I was in a taxi, rushing away from the location of one of my most memorable nights ever.

Staying inside the hotel hadn't been an option. I had to go to the training ground, as it was 8.45 already. Jordan, in the meantime, was still in bed – completely exhausted. The bed, an enormous queen-size, was situated in the £450-a-night Anchorage Suite, which had the proportions of a decent ballroom. She was sleeping off a night of wild and passionate lust, despite the fact that we both had been rat-arsed.

Nevertheless, I still remember what happened once we reached the room. Within a minute we were naked, and a few seconds later we had taken over the bed. And there we finished it off.

Sorry, guys, no footage of the action! Didn't fancy the idea of having our romp filmed. Somebody had told me she'd done a thing like that before, so once again that night I was aware of the possible presence of a candid camera.

Apart from a healthy appetite for sex, we both share a love for tattoos, Jordan and me. Nowadays it's a common thing among footballers, but back in the day I was one of the first to have himself inked. So far, there are some nice illustrations on my chest, belly, arms, hands and legs, but my back is still empty. Gotta do something about that soon.

Katie – as I should call her from now on – already had something drawn on her back: a butterfly. Beautifully done. As if he's just sneaking out of her panties, the cheeky insect. Just as nice, tattoo-wise, is the red and black heart on her, how shall we call it, 'front bottom'. Quite spectacular.

But Katie's tattoos were not what I was thinking about as I raced away in that taxi. No, the one thing on my mind was: how on earth will I get away with this?

Graciela was due back in Scotland that very day. And Graciela is not stupid. Graciela can read papers. And recognise faces in pictures. To cut a long story short, the moment she walked into International Arrivals, she saw the front page of the *Evening News*, with an enormous photo of yours truly sneaking out of the hotel. Caption: 'Fernando looked a million dollars when he arrived with Jordan, but he was like a spent penny when he left.'

'I confess,' I said to Graciela. Well, what else could I say? This: 'If Brad Pitt invited you for a hot night, you would do it too!'

Now that was a dumb thing to say. Graciela screamed that she would never do a thing like that. But I didn't believe her, so I told her again. 'Saying no to Brad Pitt would be the stupidest thing to do! All women would fall for it, especially when they've been drinking, and you're no exception!'

Very bad words, in hindsight. They made her angrier and sadder. She grabbed her suitcases, which she hadn't even opened yet, and went straight back to Glasgow Airport. Back to Alkmaar, the town she'd left just a few hours earlier.

I wouldn't see her for weeks.

I could've whacked myself. You stupid . . . But at the same time I didn't care. After all, it wasn't our first fight. Besides, with her in Alkmaar, at least I could have some fun in Glasgow again, that night. I was, as you may have noticed by now, only concerned about myself.

I never regretted my rendezvous with Katie Price. It was a real one-off, the chance of a lifetime – unlike an Old Firm match, which you can play more than once each year. Katie Price, the British Pamela Anderson . . . Every man dreams about her and only the hypocrites say they don't.

People loved the fact that I had bagged such a trophy. They congratulated me. Complete strangers would give me the thumbs-up as I walked down the street, as if I had shagged her on their behalf.

And, to be honest, it did feel like winning a major prize. So I didn't care about the resultant fine and paid the £25,000 with a smile. After all, what's a little bit of money for a night of nudity with Katie Price?

I was damn proud of myself – it really was one hell of an achievement. That's why I didn't object to the penalty. £25,000 is quite a price tag for sex, but at the same time it was an experience I will never forget. Just a pity that I left my gold bracelet at her place . . .

For months after that memorable night of pure magic we sent each other text messages on an almost daily basis. And, despite what you guys may think, it wasn't just filth and sleaze we exchanged. There was a lot of serious stuff too. About her autistic son Harvey, for instance, who suffers from Prader-Willi Syndrome.

Since then, we've only met once, at her enormous villa in Essex. It wasn't really what you'd call a success though. To be honest, at that stage I was pretty much over it with her. Novelty wears off, you know? Soon after that she moved to the Australian jungle for ITV's *I'm A Celebrity . . . Get Me Out Of Here!* And that was it.

Well, I was too busy anyway, with football and with girls.

Our last contact must have been in September 2005 when she invited me to her wedding with Peter Andre. Would be lovely to see you there, she said. Well, thanks but no thanks! What was I supposed to do there? Watch her tie the knot? Not exactly my idea of a nice day out!

We haven't talked to each other since.

Who knows how she remembers me, but I think she likes me. No, I know she likes me. And I have proof.

Three years after our romantic collision, Katie was in the Netherlands. She had been invited to a launch party for *Life After Football*, a glossy ran by former Feyenoord, Sheffield Wednesday and, yes, Celtic ace Regi Blinker. As I was in Russia at the time I couldn't be there. But in a way I was, as people were talking about me.

Robert Pot, son of my coach Cor Pot, never believed a word of my stories. So, the moment he saw Katie, this was his chance to verify what I'd been telling him all the time. So he went straight up to her, didn't even introduce himself, I believe.

Next day, he informed me how much respect he had for me, as all my antics had indeed been true. And because Katie was happy to meet 'a friend of Fernando' she stayed with him during the entire event. In the end Robert's arm must have been as blue as a Rangers shirt, as he was constantly pinching himself. According to him, everybody was after her that night but she kept sending guys away, including hot shots like Patrick Kluivert and Ruud Gullit. The only man she was interested in was Fernando Ricksen. Robert had to answer one question after the other about me.

In the end, she gave him her phone number, which, unfortunately for Robert, was to be handed over to me, just in case I wanted to call her. I never did. I was far away from Holland and the UK, in a country where the women were even more beautiful and mysterious than her!

Yes, Katie Price is a gorgeous girl, but in Russia she would be Miss Average.

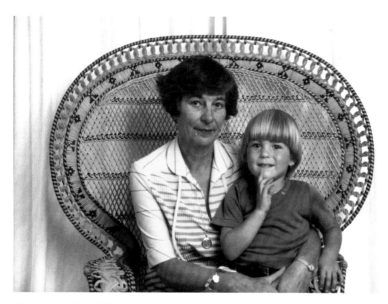

Above: Fernando with his grandmother.

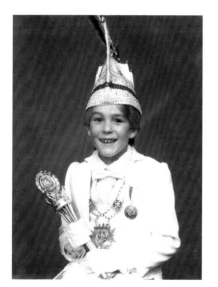

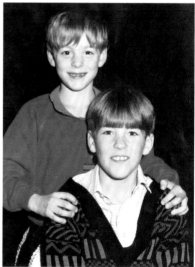

Above left: Fernando dressed as Prince Carnaval
Above right: Fernando with his brother, Pedro

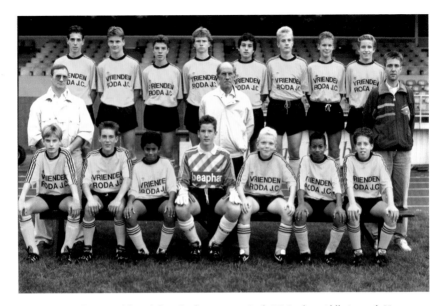

Above: Fernando, second from left in the front row, at Roda JC. In the middle is coach Hans Fischer

Below: Mark van Bommel and Fernando pose with the 1995 Eerste Divisie trophy, with Charles Vroomen, the team bus driver.

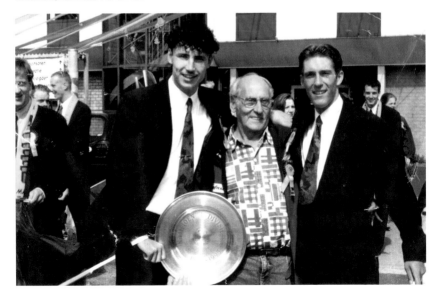

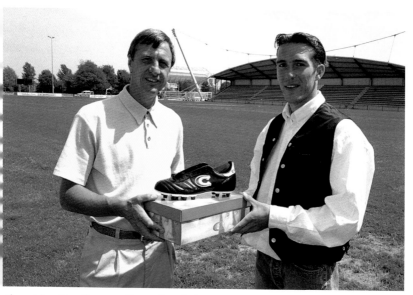

Above: Johan Cruyff presents Fernando with the 1997 Rookie of the Year award.

Below: In a duel with Dennis de Nooijer during a Fortuna Sittard-Sparta clash in 1996.

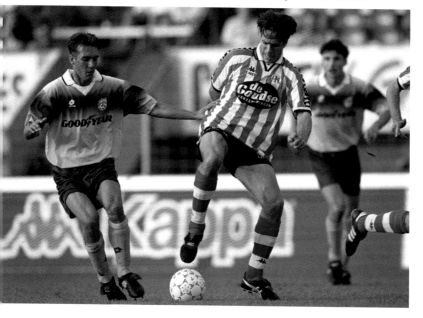

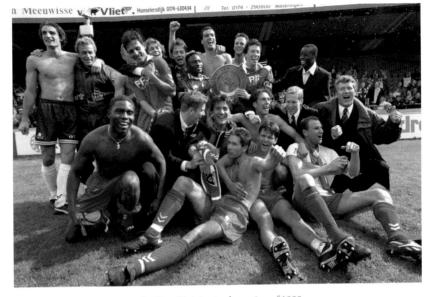

Above: AZ celebrate winning the First Division in the spring of 1998.

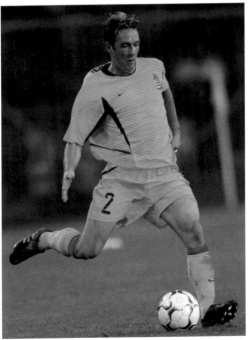

Left: Fernando in action for Holland against Portugal on 30 April, 2003, which would prove to be his last match for the national team.

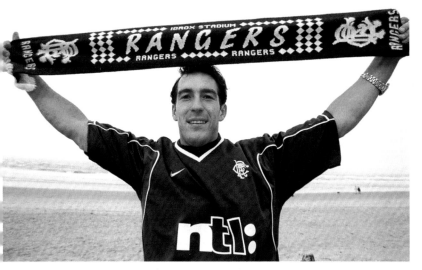

Above: Fernando celebrates signing for Rangers in March 2000.

Below: Referee Kenny Clark tries to break up a clash during the Old Firm game on 21 April, 2002; Fernando tussles with Henrik Larsson and Johan Mjallby while Arthur Numan and Lorenzo Amoruso close in to support their teammate.

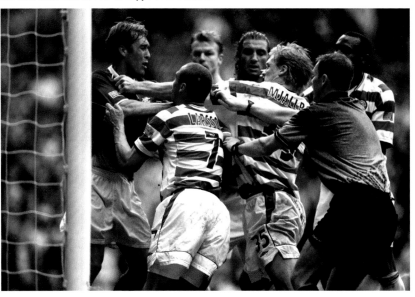

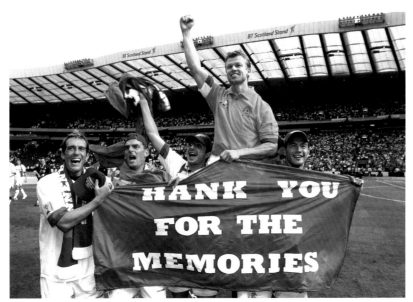

Above: Fernando, Ronald de Boer, Shota Arveladze, Arthur Numan and Michael Mols celebrate winning the Tennents Scottish Cup Final 1-0 against Dundee at Hampden Park in Glasgow, 31 May, 2003. *Getty Images*

Below: Fernando celebrates scoring in the CIS league cup final on March 20, 2005. Rangers defeated Motherwell 5-1 at Hampden Park.

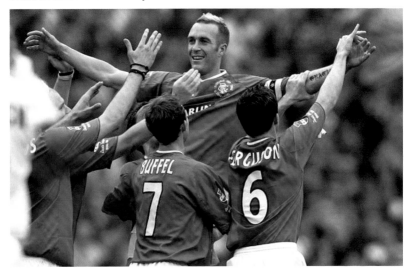

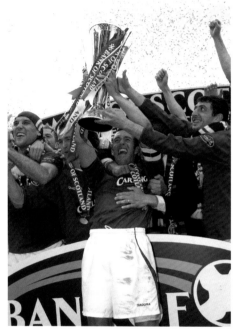

Left: Fernando lifts the Scottish Premier League trophy after defeating Hibs at Easter Road, May 22, 2005. *Getty Images*

Right: Fernando with Veronika and their daughter, Isabella.

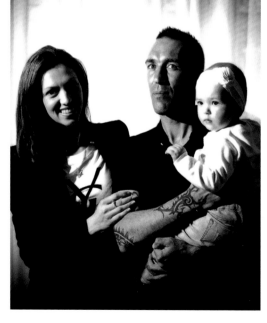

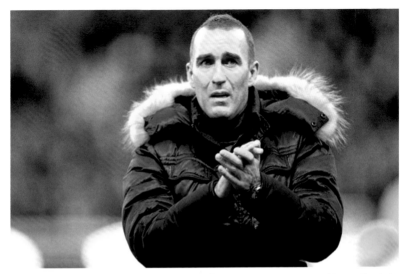

Above: Fernando makes an emotional return to Ibrox on January 11, 2014, taking to the pitch at half-time to rapturous applause during Rangers' 2-0 win over East Fife.

Below: Vincent de Vries and Fernando Ricksen, 2013.

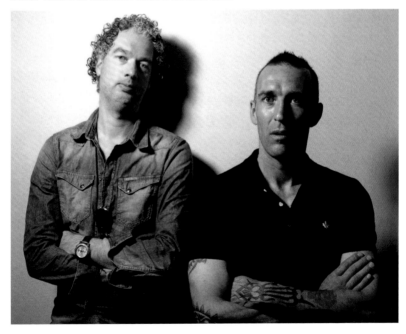

TEN

ORANGE

UNLIKE BACK HOME AT Rangers, I wasn't a top dog in the Dutch national squad. There were ten main faces, the rest were more or less hangers-on. I was one of the latter. No worries, I was just happy to be there! I could see that guys like Frank de Boer, Phillip Cocu, Jaap Stam and Edwin van der Sar had an awful lot more experience than me.

The big shots acted accordingly, as I soon found out in Huis ter Duin, the luxury hotel in the seaside village of Noordwijk where we always gathered before an international match. There wasn't actually such a thing as a hierarchy, but it was obvious that the important players made the rules. Take the seating arrangements: they made it quite clear that I couldn't just sit wherever I wanted. In order not to behave like a rebel, I always waited for the last available chair.

I almost immediately sensed a few difficulties within the group. Irritations. Lots of them rotated around Edgar Davids, an unconventional chap, it's true, although I quite liked him. The majority didn't like the fact that he kept to himself most of the time; they thought he should be more involved in group activity. Well, my view was: different characters, different habits, boys! Edgar was a loner by nature and simply wasn't a social animal like, for instance, Arthur Numan and Pierre van Hooijdonk. But did that make him a bad guy? Edgar was a phenomenal footballer – and that's what counted. Same with Clarence Seedorf. A lot of players couldn't handle his attitude, couldn't stand the fact that, despite his tender years, he always had an opinion about everything. Well, so he should, he was an incredible footballer!

The coaches didn't always like his attitude either. One day he clashed with Andries Jonker, trainee of Louis van Gaal at the national squad. But then, Jonker always acted like a schoolmaster who has to do everything by the book, so I could understand Clarence's point of view.

It was Jonker's first day as an apprentice when he said, 'Clarence, you should walk differently.'

I thought, here comes trouble! And, boy, was I right.

Seedorf, undisputedly world-class at that time, couldn't believe his ears. So he went towards this snotty kid – who was actually older than him but looked younger – and asked him who he was.

'My name's Andries Jonker.'

'Aha. Played any football yourself?'

'Eh, yes.'

'At the top?'

Jonker shook his head.

'Then shut up, will ya?'

And off he went, the only Dutch footballer who would win four Champions Leagues. But not before telling Jonker that he shouldn't forget to put the plastic cones on the training field 'as far away from us as possible, please!'

(To his credit, in 2014 Andries Jonker would end up as head of Arsenal's youth division.)

I never found out why, at a certain moment, coaches decided to leave Clarence Seedorf out of the Dutch squad. Maybe they felt threatened by the enormous amount of knowledge the kid had. But it's a shame. He ended up with a lousy 87 caps and should have had at least 150.

I liked him, from the moment we met at the under-16s in 1991. However, I didn't think I was the right person to mediate between

Clarence and the staff, all those years later. After all, at the time I had some personal problems of my own to deal with.

The Dutch press weren't an issue. Compared to the British hellhounds they were as innocent as newborn babies. As I drove my vehicle into the parking lot at Huis ter Duin, I would see them waiting in line, ready to grab the odd quote. And every time I thought to myself, aren't they cute? What a bunch of sweetie pies! They're so harmless in Holland that I came to view my Orange trips as some kind of relaxation.

Another advantage: I always had a room to myself. Fantastic, in terms of preparation. After dinner, at seven, we used to stay downstairs for a bit of a chat, but in order not to get into trouble I was always back in my room way before eleven. It was a room with a lovely sea view too.

This big private room was proof of the fact that the Dutch national team meant world-class. With Rangers, we always had to share a room. I didn't like it at all. With Zenit Saint Petersburg, Dick Advocaat managed to change that. Thank God, as I was about to share yet another room with my Turkish teammate Fatih Tekke, who had the habit of jumping out of bed at six in the morning to pray. Afterwards, he would light a cigarette and watch TV, which drove me insane.

No praying or snoring roommates in Huis ter Duin. No filthy hacks either, just a bunch of well-behaved Dutch reporters. It was always the same, on the steps leading to the hotel. They'd ask me a few standard questions, I'd give them a few standard answers and that was that. They were happy with it. Well, happy to be of service, gentlemen!

I didn't act like a rebel within the national squad. Why would I? And how could I? The big boss was Louis van Gaal, Mr Discipline. Well, let me tell you: no one messes with him!

Apart from being Mr Discipline, he is also Mr Perfection, as Pierre van Hooijdonk found out.

Now, Pierre doesn't like to wear socks. Inside his shoes, he's always barefoot. So there he was, one morning in 2001, in the

Sheraton Hotel at Schiphol Airport, a few days before our game against Andorra – without the obligatory white socks. When Van Gaal noticed this fashion statement he exploded. '*That is not the agreement!*' And, believe me, the man can shout. (Little did he know that poor Pierre had almost shown up without wearing a tie either. Fixed it at the last moment in the elevator.)

But it wasn't about bullying people. Van Gaal wanted us to be a united team. Only then can one achieve great things.

He always wanted the maximum amount of commitment and concentration from us. Mistakes were not tolerated. If you did something wrong, you were humiliated.

Here's an example for you. Ronald Waterreus, my Rangers teammate, always did the goal kicks. He was brilliant at it. Left foot, right foot, perfect! I swear I've never seen anyone as good as him. Until, for no reason, one kick went completely wrong and the ball ended up near the corner flag. Just an accident, but Van Gaal wasn't impressed.

'*This is the goddamn national team, Waterreus! If you can't manage to kick a ball in a straight line you better go home!*'

I was shocked. So all these stories about Van Gaal were true. But how? The guy must have eyes in the back of his head, I mused. He'd been facing away from the action at the time.

It made me insecure, to tell you the truth. Louis van Gaal meant the utmost professionalism, and I wasn't used to that yet. Mind you, two years earlier I was still playing in the Dutch First Division. But, no excuses, mate! The man wanted you to be part of his squad, so you better not disappoint him.

Still, as I was now playing with Holland's best footballers, I was a bit confused. Should I play like I always did at Rangers? I didn't want to hurt the likes of Seedorf and De Boer. Play tough, don't play tough? I didn't know what to do. And, as it happened, I was using my brains more than my feet. All in all, not much came of it.

Van Gaal noticed immediately. After the training session he took me aside, put an arm around my shoulder and said, 'Fernando, I fully understand that you're nervous. Just one word of advice: do as you always do at your club. Do your own thing. Don't compromise. Don't do a little bit of this and a little bit of that, okay?'

We shook hands and I promised not to disappoint him.

More than anything else, it was the speed at which the guys played. It was so much faster than I was used to. After the first Orange training, I was totally exhausted and went straight to bed. I didn't even have the energy to turn on the TV.

But Van Gaal's encouraging words had an enormous impact on me. The next day I felt a lot more relaxed, and not as tired afterwards. I was on the way up.

Not a bad word about LVG from my side. The man is a phenomenon, a remarkable manager who always manages to get the best out of a player. You have to work damn hard, that's for sure, but the end result always lives up to his expectations. Like no other – with the possible exception of Advocaat – he can make you better. And eventually you become just as fanatical as he is. A true craftsman!

As I didn't want to screw things up – I was too damn proud of my orange shirt – I refused to hit the bottle once I was in Holland. Playing for the national team had been a childhood dream, so I was definitely not going to blow it. I still remember that day in Glasgow in 2000 when Dick Advocaat told me he had received a phone call from the Dutch FA, the KNVB. Van Gaal wanted me to play against Ireland, on 15 November in Amsterdam. World Cup qualification, phew! I was more than a little surprised, especially as things weren't really hitting a crescendo at Rangers.

Later on, driving back to Newton Mearns, I had a smile the width of a football goal. Suddenly I saw a lot of possibilities. Fact: I was far from my best at Rangers. Yet, I had qualified as one of the best eighteen footballers in my country. So, I said to myself, 'What will happen the moment you do play well at the club?' I was convinced I was going to be a regular then. A comforting thought, given that the World Cup in Japan and South Korea was only two years away.

Unfortunately I wouldn't play a single minute against Ireland. Even when right-winger Michael Reiziger was injured I had to stay on the bench. We were a goal down, thanks to a shot by Robbie Keane, so van Gaal chose a more experienced substitute, one with a strong desire to attack. So it was Clarence Seedorf in my spot, and Paul Bosvelt had to shift backwards. Half an hour before the end of the game, Jason McAteer scored – 0–2 – and I knew I would be a spectator for the rest of the night. Well, at least Jeffrey Talan and Giovanni van Bronckhorst made it 2–2, but it wasn't enough for me to save the evening. I kept my orange shirt, but it was a small consolation.

One month later, there was the double confrontation with Cyprus and Portugal and, yes, once again I was part of the squad! It was a huge relief, I can tell you, especially because I still wasn't doing well at Rangers. At the least, a few days away from Scotland would be relaxing.

Relaxing? Au contraire! One day before the match against Cyprus, I was injured. Even worse, I ended up in a wheelchair! So once again I had to experience the game as part of the crowd.

It was my ankle, the same ankle that was damaged all those years ago by PSV's Ernest Faber. And it was double trouble, as thanks to the injury I didn't miss one, but two international games! My replacement, Mario Melchiot, couldn't have had a better week.

Anyway, I'm not the kind of person to be stopped just like that. Five weeks later I was back playing for the mighty Orange. We had to face Spain in a friendly in Seville. I came on as a substitute, aged 24 (and 111 days, for the Stattos among you). Just as I had predicted, I had made my debut in the national team before my twenty-fifth birthday.

Take that, Chris Dekker!

Yes, I was a substitute, as Van Gaal wanted to play things safe. It was a month after a painful defeat against Portugal, so tensions were pretty high. The only new player who could start immediately was Kevin Hofland. Me and my old pal Patrick Paauwe – of that hotel incident with the chicks – started on the bench.

Thirty minutes into the second half, I started my warm-up: the usual stretching and stuff, which I normally hate. Just let me get rid of my training jacket and I'll run straight onto the pitch for you, no problem at all. But this was the national team and this was Louis van Gaal, so for a change I did exactly what I was told.

It was 1–1, with goals from Fernando Hierro and Jimmy 'Floyd' Hasselbaink. With fifteen minutes to go, Van Gaal sensed we could win. And it showed. The man was screaming his lungs out, acting as if he personally wanted to score. Great to see. Five minutes to go. A header by Frank de Boer. 1–2!

More important, I was sent on as a replacement for Paul Bosvelt! Okay, it was just for a few minutes, but I was in the Dutch national team! And look who I was facing. Iker Casillas! Carles Puyol! Xavi! Raúl! Luis Enrique!

I was impressed, but I couldn't show it. Not now. I had to stay focused more than ever. No way was I going to screw this up!

The first ball I got came from the foot of Michael Reiziger. Too slow, not enough speed; it hardly reached me. One moment I was thinking, Why is he giving me such a lousy pass? The next moment I was on the grass screaming.

Sergi had hit my ankle. Merciless.

'How are you, Fernando?' It was the voice of the doctor. I was still on the ground, and our medic was trying to revive me.

'I'm fine,' I lied.

Of course I wasn't. I was in more agony than I could handle. It hurt like hell. That bastard, Sergi! What did he think this was? A Champions League Final? It was just a friendly!

Determined not to leave the pitch, I got up after three minutes – for a total of two seconds. End of the game.

The next four weeks, in Glasgow, my ankle was wrapped in plastic filled with ice cubes. I didn't mind. I was just happy that I'd made it into our national team. I had a cap. A virtual one, as in Holland they don't really hand those things out, but still.

For a while, my international career was limited to those few seconds against Spain. In 2001 I didn't play at all. My problems in Glasgow had worsened and they got way too big for me to be selected again. First, get yourself back on track again, was the message van Gaal gave me. Not easy to hear, but he was right. Now it was up to me to show the whole world that I wasn't just a one-hit wonder.

By 2002 I was doing well again in Scotland, but things had changed in and around the Dutch national team. After failing to qualify for the World Cup van Gaal was given his marching orders. Sad for him, but not so much for me, as his successor was one Dick Advocaat! Yup, the very man who knew everything about me. The one who, like no other, was familiar with my Fighting Spirit.

Come February 2002 and there I was again, in a friendly against our English neighbours. Their squad read like a who's who of British football: David Beckham, Frank Lampard, Steven Gerrard, Rio Ferdinand, Paul Scholes . . .

I was beaming. Now *this* promised to be a great game! I could hardly wait.

And thanks to Dick I could start from minute one. It felt like an enormous victory – a victory over myself.

The moment I walked onto the pitch, surrounded by thousands of lads dressed in orange, was one of the happiest moments of my life. And I've felt the same in every single match since then. I know, I'm not like Frank de Boer who has 112 caps. Fat chance he remembers every one of those games though. I have 100 less, 767 minutes in total, but I can tell you who scored in every match and what every goal looked like.

Proud as a peacock when I walked on the pitch, proud as a peacock when I left it. It was a great game, although it ended in a 1–1 draw due to goals by Patrick Kluivert and Darius Vassell. At least I had shown the world that I was back! Thanks to my direct opponent Emile Heskey for being so big and strong. I like players like this particular Liverpool forward. Don't fancy the small ones, as proven in my Old Firm matches with Bobby Petta.

Stay focused now, I told myself, that memorable night in Amsterdam. Don't do anything stupid. Don't screw it up.

But I did screw it up – big time – thanks to that old devil called booze. My career as an international would reach as far as a strip joint in the city of Minsk.

But that's another chapter.

ELEVEN

LIFE SENTENCE

EVERY TIME I WAS invited to play for the national team, my self-esteem got a boost. Not that I was one of the top boys by then; I knew my place. Still, my self-confidence was growing – to the point where I was courageous enough to play the odd prank. Until then I'd only tried to be funny at AZ and Rangers! It was the support I got from Dick Advocaat which increased my self-confidence, just as it had at, yup, AZ and Rangers.

I was getting closer to a lot of the main guys. Apart from those I knew from my Fortuna and Rangers days, it was mainly the black guys I ended up rubbing shoulders with. They had their own group within the squad, but I didn't see why I couldn't join them. After all, they could see I wasn't exactly dull, and I remembered a few of them from my youth too. Like Patrick Kluivert.

We spent a lot of time together talking – and not just about football. A lot had happened to him in previous years, from the high of scoring the winning goal in the Champions League Final in 1995 to killing a man in a car crash just a few months later. Without wanting to sound like a would-be therapist, I sensed Patrick enjoyed our chats.

We were getting along so well that we even teamed up in Newcastle, where he was playing for the local pride. Now, the Geordie capital wasn't new to me – I'd been there a few times already. Brilliant city! Just like Liverpool and Manchester. Perfect cities for a good night out – and all within travelling distance from Glasgow. Newcastle has been dubbed the Party Capital of the UK – and the title is well earned! Every time I jumped into my car to race to the banks of the river Tyne I impersonated a Smiley for the entire journey.

We shared a lot of interests, Patrick and me, so when Dick, right after the Euro 2004 qualification match against Belarus, in June 2003, told us we could go out to celebrate the last international game of the season, we both thought the same. This would be a night to remember!

Of course, I'd done my homework. I knew that Belarus was home to the most beautiful women in the world.

Dick, bless him, told us we could stay out for as long as we wanted. 'Only one thing, guys: tomorrow at nine we have a bus heading for the airport. If you're late, we won't wait.'

No problem, Dick!

Nine o'clock in the morning . . . sounds a bit early, doesn't it? So it came in handy that I already knew where the nearest strip joint was. Inside the hotel building! In the basement, to be precise. No idea whether the Dutch FA was aware of it when they booked the hotel, but what did I care? This was brilliant, absolutely brilliant!

The game itself, you ask? Well, I didn't play. Michael Reiziger was back – in more ways than one! That was a bit of a pity, but no more than that. The fact is, I was still recuperating from a couple of very heavy nights. You see, the previous Saturday we had won the SFA Cup and because of that we'd been partying like animals. *Noblesse oblige!*

Other than my fellow Ranger Ronald de Boer, who had also been selected for the game in Minsk, I didn't get an extra day off from Dick. It was straight to the players' hotel on Monday. But then, when I arrived in Noordwijk, I noticed there were only eight players in total! All the guys had been enjoying a nice weekend off, while I had a Cup Final in my legs! That, and two nights of heavy drinking. Not fair, eh?

Fast-forward to the game in Minsk. That was an easy one: a 2–0 victory, with goals by Marc Overmars and Patrick Kluivert. Due to the result we were still in the race for Euro 2004 in Portugal.

For me, it was a different game to the usual. Normally, when sitting on the bench, I would be focused on my direct rival. I would analyse every single one of his movements and ball contacts. This time I was only thinking about the strippers in the cellar.

Back in my hotel room, I threw my bag on the floor, and within minutes me and a few teammates were sitting in a taxi. Yup, first we went out. Of course we went out! Why shouldn't we? Because we're football players and therefore role models? People who condemn us for painting the town red are hypocrites. They're allowed to do so and we shouldn't be? Bollocks! Footballers are human beings!

More from the Department of Hypocrisy: I can't stand footballers who deny it when they've been on the piss. You know, guys with a stomach but without balls. Grow up! Either don't go, or go and admit it. I've done a lot of things that I maybe shouldn't have done, but after being caught I've always pleaded guilty.

Notwithstanding this: not being caught was my main concern. And, hell, that was difficult in the UK! The tabloid press is like a giant octopus with enormous tentacles. Ask Arthur Numan, that cheerful chap from the lovely town of Beverwijk. Kissed a girl in a bar, as you do. Totally innocent stuff. But poor old Arthur hadn't noticed the CCTV camera above his head. Too engrossed, perhaps. The next morning we found out that CCTV stuff is sometimes sold to newspapers. King Arthur must have been hiding under his round table for the rest of the day!

So I was always careful – very careful. For instance, there's only one picture of me and Jordan together. One! Bobby took it and, no, we're not going to show it to you!

I really chose my spots for a well-deserved snog. Like the loo. Lesson one: never jump into them together! Always let the girl come a few minutes after you, otherwise it's way too obvious. Nevertheless, I sometimes wish I had done certain things a bit differently. Like, you've guessed it, that night in Minsk.

Because the open-air disco in town was a bit disappointing, we went back to the hotel quite early. Back to bed. Well, most of the lads did. I stayed up. After all, there was this basement that needed to be inspected.

It was paradise, pure paradise . . .

I noticed it the moment I entered the place. Top models galore! So I decided to stay for as long as possible. And to celebrate that decision I started to pamper my inner self with alcohol. Lots of it.

Thanks to a drinking binge of many, many hours, I completely lost sense of time and space. I thought I was even hallucinating as I swear I felt Willem van Hanegem tapping me on the shoulder and saying, 'You better get ready, pal. It's five to nine and the bus is about to leave.'

Oh shit!

It *was* Willem van Hanegem! Well, of course it was. My former AZ coach was now Dick's assistant at the national team. But, wait, this meant . . . *I had five minutes to collect my stuff and get to the airport bus!*

So, it was a quick goodbye to the girls and an even quicker run to the room – together with my partner in crime, Patrick Kluivert, who had been with me all those drink-sodden hours.

Within two minutes I reached my room. *On schedule!* A few seconds to grab my bag and three full minutes to go down the elevator and reach the bus – that shouldn't be too much of a problem. So . . . *shit, shit, shit, shit!* My door key, one of those plastic swipecards, wouldn't work! It had been inside my trouser pocket for most of the evening, and it was now battered and folded.

I tried it again, sweat pouring down my face. Still not!

The bus was going to leave without me! And the plane! Or would they? Nah, they would wait for me. Would they? Maybe not! Better not wait to find out, Fernando!

There was hardly a minute left. Not enough time to go down to the reception and ask for a new swipecard. I made a split-second decision. I thought to myself: what is it that you do best? The answer was, obviously, kicking. So I took a run and . . . *kicked the entire door in!*

The next thing I saw was Ruud van Nistelrooy, ready to go down with his bag, looking as if he'd seen a ghost. 'Your room is next to mine, pal,' he said.

I'd demolished the wrong door!

By now, time was *really* running out, so I decided to – well, it's obvious really – kick in my own door too! Two doors in a few seconds. That's Belarus carpentry for you.

It never occurred to me that, together with the doors, I was kicking my international career to pieces. Well, there wasn't time for contemplation. All that counted was: grab bag, race to bus!

But racing wasn't an option. I was totally plastered. I was moving sideways as well as straight ahead. Van Hanegem had to grab me at one point, otherwise I would have fallen flat on my face. As I got on the bus, I acted as if I had just woken up. But I'm not exactly Sean Connery.

Dick saw straight away I was drunk – and he didn't like what he saw. Believe it or not, I was even a bit insulted by his reaction. What the hell? I was on time, wasn't I?

To make things worse, the moment we entered the airport, I went straight to the bar to order a beer and gulped it down in a few seconds. As I threw the fizzy stuff down my throat Dick Advocaat walked by. He looked straight into my blood-red eyes and I knew he was close to exploding.

The next day, as I told the guys about my antics, my fellow Rangers were in stitches. I, on the other hand, wasn't exactly proud of what I'd done in Minsk. Somebody told me I'd drunk out of a flower vase. Now that's something I wish hadn't happened . . . One thing was clear: I had fucked things up. Completely, this time.

Two months later, before a friendly against Belgium, I wasn't part of the Dutch side any more. At least Dick had the guts to tell me in person. He didn't have a choice, he said over the phone. I fully understood. Not punishing me would have made him the wrong man for the job. I told him that I didn't find it fair that he just castigated me – and not any of the others. 'Fernando,' he said, 'what you did was way out of control. It was unbelievable. As a professional football organisation we can't tolerate this kind of behaviour. I'm sure you'll understand.'

Well, I had to. I couldn't force him to let me play, could I?

It was a life sentence. My Orange days were over. After Belgium Holland played against Austria, the Czech Republic, Moldova and even, in the play-offs, Scotland. Every single game without me.

So, instead of playing in Portugal, in the summer of 2004, I was on a beach somewhere on the other side of the globe. Didn't enjoy it. I was beaten to a pulp – by myself.

I would never receive another invitation for an international game. The only thing the Dutch FA sent me was a bill for two new doors. For the association, that incident had been the umpteenth in a short spell. One year prior to my booze-fuelled madness, there had been a skirmish near a pub in Oslo, shortly after we'd played a Norway away game, although on that particular occasion I wasn't the centre of attention. It was Jimmy 'Floyd' Hasselbaink, salesman in goals.

We had been told there was a nice boozer within walking distance of our hotel. So we decided to pay it a visit. When in Norway, drink as the Norwegians do, or so they say. I've no idea whether it was a nice boozer or not, as we never made it past the door.

Hasselbaink was refused admittance. Because he's black? I honestly can't tell you, but the fact is that the bouncers refused entry to the only black guy in our group. That meant a lot of yelling, cursing, pushing, pulling . . . and flashing, as a Scandinavian photographer tried to capture the whole scene on camera. I still don't know how many real punches were thrown – if any – but there was a lot of commotion, I can tell you.

To avoid the whole thing escalating, we marched back to our hotel. Case closed, as far as we were concerned. But not so for the Dutch FA. Our security man Bertus Holkema was fired after the incident. Too bad, as we liked the guy. Okay, his task was to prevent us from getting bad press and, yes, it was him who had taken us into town, but still . . .

For the football association it was simply a matter of 'too much, too often'. After all, they were still dealing with the aftermath of the Kira Eggers incident.

Kira Eggers! Now that's a name that rings a bell among Dutch football fans . . . Kira Eggers, Danish escort girl cum porn star (or the other way around), had sneaked into the players' hotel, together with a few of her curvy colleagues, just hours before the match against Denmark. According to eyewitnesses (and the press), it went off there and then. And Louis van Gaal didn't like it when he read about it. Nor did the Dutch FA.

Unfortunately I was injured at the time, as I would love to have met Miss Eggers. Checked her on the internet later. Tasty! Anyway, I wasn't surprised when I heard the stories about Kinky Kira. After all, she wasn't the first female predator who'd made her way into our settlement. I never forget the hours after my debut against Spain. The corridors of our hotel were packed with giggling girls. I was used to this kind of thing at Rangers, but, hey, this was a national team, a bunch of people representing their country!

Still, I didn't do anything naughty back then. It was my first time with the squad, so I didn't want to lose all my credits. Yet. But I was pissed off, I can tell you! Why on earth wasn't I involved? Just gimme a call and I'll come, quite literally. It's not that I was bothered by small details like the fact that it was the evening before an international match!

Oh, and please don't feed me that bullshit about sex before a game! That it isn't good for an athlete and stuff. If I may speak for myself, I needed it! It made me perform better. It took the pressure off. Don't forget there's a lot of a weight on a professional footballer's shoulders. What, for instance, do you think happens when a player has to take a penalty? The pressure is immense. People really underestimate that. The idea that millions and millions of eyes are staring at you causes enormous tension. You have to be able to cope with that, otherwise things fall apart – especially when you realise that your kick can make the difference between fifteen million euros and a few hundred grand. That stress, I can tell you, is unbearable. It was also the reason why teammates of mine were snorting cocaine and downing pills on a regular basis. It was a way to handle the tension.

Talking about being kicked out of the squad, Dick wouldn't be the last one to do that to me. In 2006, McLeish's successor at Rangers, Paul Le Guen, told me he didn't need me any more. I was speechless when I heard it. I didn't know the man and he didn't know me, so this was not something I'd expected. Hence the optimistic mood in which I entered his room. I had been Rangers' captain, Player of the Year, figurehead, so surely he was going to discuss next season's plans with his most valuable player. Not quite!

'I have bad news for you,' was his opening line. 'Very bad news.' The man didn't show any emotion as he continued. 'You can search for another club. In my plans, there is no room for you.'

I couldn't believe my ears. In my mind I cursed him. But more than that I asked myself: why, why, why? Didn't he see how important I was? Didn't he see how popular I was? Didn't he see how many fans were wearing a shirt with my name? Didn't he want to see how important and popular I was? Was it the language? The strange thing with this Frenchman was that he didn't speak English at all. Not a single word. He spoke via an interpreter. Always! Didn't look you in the eyes either. A real weirdo, in my opinion.

Still, I managed to stay calm. Told him that he was possibly drawing his conclusions a bit too quickly. 'Give it a month, boss. You don't even know me yet.' I told him he would really need me. 'Boss, this is Scotland. Here, things don't go the way they do in the rest of Europe. You can't survive without players like me. Believe me, this is going to be your downfall. Without me you'll be gone within six months. No doubt about it.'

Le Guen wasn't having any of it. It seemed as if he had only one thing on his mind: exterminate Ricksen! 'I simply don't want you,' he let his translator say. The one thing he didn't need his ventriloquist dummy for was to point at the door.

Well, the message was clear. I had to go. Now, up to that point I'd dealt with the odd disappointment, but this was a real blow. And all that was left for me to do was guess. Why was he so eager to get rid of me? Maybe because he couldn't bear the idea of having big stars on the pitch. They would be a threat to a mediocre manager like him.

From that moment on he started to humiliate me, treated me like a rookie. Expelled me from the first team and put me into the second. Le Guen was aiming to break me. And even worse: he succeeded.

Away went my support in life. Away went my structure. From that moment on, I grew more and more depressed. I stayed at home, didn't go out any more. The fact that I'd lost the most precious thing in life, being an important footballer at an important club, turned me into a recluse. And, worse of all, I didn't even care. Back home I started to hit the bottle more and more. And that led to some dangerous situations. Because I couldn't sleep I would drink myself unconscious.

Looking back now, I realise I shouldn't have done that. Instead, I should have showed my Fighting Spirit. But at the time I couldn't. All I thought was: screw you, Le Guen. In six months' time you'll be dead meat!

So, it came as a huge surprise when I was invited to join Rangers on their training trip to South Africa in July. Somebody had dropped out at the last moment and Le Guen decided to give me a chance. Or at least that's what he said to others; I didn't communicate with the man.

At the airport I bought a big bottle of port. I didn't even hide it. I told the club doctor that I needed it to get to sleep. After all, it was a thirteen-hour flight to Johannesburg. But I'd lied. I just wanted to drink, full stop. The doc didn't like the idea and gave me sleeping pills instead. I promised to swallow them immediately. This time I didn't lie: I took the drugs. But I took the liquor as well. And that's a lethal combination at an altitude of 50,000 feet!

Next thing I know, I flipped out. I got undressed and started running up the aisles. Naked. I'd completely lost it. I even managed to pour a glass of water over a flight steward. Or so they told me afterwards. I couldn't remember. And that wasn't the only incident on that flight!

Earlier on, I had had a bit of a squabble with a stewardess about the sound level of my laptop, on which I was watching a porn flick. I think it was my teammates who kept turning up the volume, but it was definitely me and me alone who downed the pills and drank the booze. There's no one else to blame.

'You're on the next flight back,' said Le Guen, shortly after we'd landed in Johannesburg. He never wanted to see me again.

I was close to laughing when he told me to piss off. I couldn't care less; he didn't like me anyway. The thought that I would never play a game for Rangers again didn't even cross my mind. I was too far gone.

Mind you, it wasn't a totally wasted trip. Not at all. Due to the fact that the next flight home wasn't until the following day, I had an overnight stay in Jo'burg. Away from the squad, as Le Guen really didn't want to see my face any more. Instead, I was taken to an airport hotel for my own (and others') safety, so that the club doctor could keep an eye on me. I didn't mind. He was a good guy, that doc. We even did the conga that night, in an Italian restaurant, after Italy beat France in the 2006 World Cup Final. Yup, the same tournament that I would have been in if I hadn't destroyed two hotel doors.

No, it wasn't the thought of missing out on a World Cup that kept me awake that night in my South African hotel room, it was my pulsating penis. I was horny as hell – and that needed to be fixed. I jumped out of bed, grabbed the newspaper that I had found in the lobby, and started checking the escort agency ads.

I rang the first number I saw and asked for a black girl. No problem, they said. She would be 'there in half an hour'. I could pick her up at reception.

Not long after, while I was lying in the arms of my lover, there was a knock on the door.

'Yes?' I asked.

'It's me.' It was the doctor. And he sounded worried.

'Fernando, are you in bed already?'

'Yes!' I screamed in all honesty. And to prove that I wasn't lying,

I walked to the door and opened it. Naked. 'But I'm not alone,' I grinned.

The doc was stretching like a ballerina to try to get a glimpse of my bed partner. 'Just,' he mumbled, 'make sure that you're not too late tomorrow morning.'

'No worries,' I said. And I went back to finish what I'd started.

Rangers, on the other hand, were finishing things too. I received a phone call a few hours later from my new agent, Rob Jansen, who told me that my situation at the club had become untenable. 'We really have to find you a new club, Fernando.'

Another call I got was from Peter Kay, director of the Sporting Chance Clinic and an acquaintance of McLeish. 'Forget about football for the moment, Fernando,' he said to me, sounding really concerned. 'Just get to our clinic in Hampshire straight away.' Now that didn't sound like an unreasonable idea. Rangers wouldn't make a big fuss out of it, as alcohol addiction is almost a Scottish disease. 'We can help you, Fernando,' Kay continued. 'I can't force you to go to the clinic, but as a friend I would like to say to you: grab my hand. Otherwise, believe me, it's over. You're in serious trouble, Fernando.'

So there he was, this man, thousands of miles away, telling me about the things this special clinic for sportsmen had to offer. I was told they had ways of getting fellow fallen heroes off gambling, drugs, sex and alcohol.

But I was sceptical. I wasn't an addict. I was a social drinker. Up until then I had never even thought about rehab. I could do without booze – for days, if needed! Okay, after a dry spell there was always a bit of a relapse, but, still, I could handle things myself perfectly well. Or so I thought.

But during Kay's phone call in that Jo'burg hotel, it suddenly dawned on me: I had lost it. Completely. And I couldn't continue like this. All the lies, the cheating, the double-crossing . . . I wasn't even being honest with myself. Kay was right: I was killing myself. And I did have to check in to the clinic, I had to! Not so much for the drinking as such, but more for the problems it caused. It had to stop. I was – literally! – in the Last Chance Saloon.

'I'm on my way,' I said to Kay. And I meant it.

So, instead of fighting for my last chance at Rangers, on a football field in South Africa, I was fighting for my last chance in life, in a medical centre in England.

The flight to Johannesburg had been a bumpy one, but it turned out to be my lifesaver.

TWELVE

RELIEF

THE DRIVE TO THE clinic in Liphook, about 37 miles from London, didn't take long. From Heathrow it took about an hour. I didn't say much during the journey despite the cab driver being up for some chit-chat. I was thinking about what I'd done. Finally. Thinking about the mess I'd made of my life.

Suddenly it dawned on me that I hadn't taken enough clothes with me. It was basically just football gear and a bit of leisurewear, as I'd flown straight from South Africa. There was no time to go home first, they had told me. This was urgent.

The clinic itself was a beauty. The lakeside setting, in the South Downs National Park, was impressive, to say the least. It was also interesting that Arsenal's Tony Adams, the Gunner-turned-Gulper, had given his name and blessing to the institution. Thanks to the twilight, the place looked like a fairytale castle. It had a never-ending driveway without a single lamppost. This was deliberate, the staff later told me, to minimise the risk of people doing a runner. They would get lost in the dark – and that wasn't a pleasant idea.

Not that I was thinking about escaping when I was sitting in the backseat of the taxi. Oh no. Still, if I did fancy the idea of running away, I could do it. Piece of cake. After all, I'd done it on numerous occasions with Rangers . . .

The *Escape from Alcatraz* planning began the moment we entered the hotel car park. Sitting in the players' coach I was already looking at the possibilities: 'Mmmm, drainpipe next to the window . . .'

That was why I always wanted a room at the front of the hotel. 'On the lowest available floor, thank you.'

If I wasn't provided with the room of my choice, I'd swap with a teammate, especially if he was a youngster. After all, those kids didn't care where they slept. And they wouldn't say no to Big Fernando.

I never sneaked out on my own. Most of the time I was joined by some of the usual suspects, like Thomas Buffel. Once, in Toronto for a training camp, we even managed to use our lunch break to go to a strip joint! Being one hell of a tour guide, I'd found out in advance that there was one just across the road. 'We're going for a walk,' we said, after the morning training had finished. The coaches agreed, but little did they know . . .

So, while the rest of the team were having their post-training cuppa, the two of us, immaculately attired in our tracksuits, were enjoying the sight of naked bodies wrapped around a pole. A bit of stretching, boss!

Evenings were never spent in front of the TV or over a game of Trivial Pursuit. Out through the in-door we went – if we were sure the manager was asleep. It was always the same pattern. Take taxi. Visit strip club. Watch clock. Because, above anything else, we had to be back before breakfast. Just imagine the manager enjoying his coffee and morning paper and suddenly he catches sight of his players sneaking in to the hotel . . . Not the best guarantee for a place in the next match!

I'm sure our technical superiors were aware of our off-the-pitch antics anyway. Not least because a lot of them were enthusiastic drinkers too. I remember Andy Watson, McLeish's loyal assistant, sleeping it off in the corridor of a New York hotel. Dick Advocaat, then technical director, saw him and just shook his head as he walked past the intoxicated body.

Okay, so we weren't what you might call ascetics. But, one thing I can assure you, when we were training, the fact that we'd been drinking all night never showed. Never! To an outsider we looked as clean and fresh as, well, a group of athletes. More to the point, we pushed ourselves even harder. In order not to be discovered as pissheads, we trained at 150 per cent, maybe even more! We worked harder and were more fanatical than under normal circumstances. I felt sorry for the young kids who had gone to bed early, probably with a hot cocoa, and now had to suffer for the dirty deeds of a bunch of alcoholics.

So, there I was in the English clinic thinking: if I really want to escape, I can. Definitely. For instance, during my wee hour of cycling every morning. It wouldn't be too difficult to turn that into a mini-Tour de France. Bye, Tony Adams, I'll send you a postcard!

But the truth is: I didn't want to. I sort of liked the place. It wasn't exactly a prison. It was more like a health resort, so why not stay there for the full four weeks? Besides, I could stop this therapy whenever I wanted. It was all on a voluntary basis. So, technically speaking, 'escape' wasn't even the right verb.

The only thing we didn't have at the clinic was a television. Like so many other things, that was deliberate. We weren't to receive any stimulation from the outside world: that was the idea behind it. Sometimes I peeped into the room of the medics, as they were allowed to watch TV themselves, but the moment they saw me they sent me away, like I was six years old.

No laptops either. That was understandable, given the stuff I used mine for on the Johannesburg flight . . .

So, I loved it there. Nobody was nagging me: perfect! No more Graciela, no more Le Guen. Well, not that the latter was thinking about me anyway. To him, I simply didn't exist any more, but I think we've been through that already.

Oh, and no journalists for a while! Now *that* was a blessing! A great country, Scotland, but its tabloids . . . The way they'd follow you wherever you went, day in, day out. Snapped in the supermarket buying a bottle of wine as a present for somebody and they'd write a story about my being on the booze again. It was hard to swallow sometimes.

So, none of that during my stay in Hampshire. And even if people did want to get in touch with me, they couldn't! You see, as I checked in, I had to hand over my phone. And they searched me to see whether I was carrying any alcohol. I thought that was a bit strange. Why on earth would I take a bottle of booze to rehab? Hey, I wasn't an alcoholic! At least not yet.

Contrary to popular belief, I wasn't as much a sponge as George Best or Paul Gascoigne. As I pointed out earlier – or didn't I? – I am not George II or This Year's Gazza. Now I've heard stories of the latter... Bobby once told me how Paul visited his restaurant in Glasgow with the sole intention of drinking the place dry. Now at a certain moment, the guy is full. And I mean: full! So what happens? The Drowning Magpie goes to the loo, sticks one of his fingers down his throat and puts the entire engine into reverse. So after his Niagara Falls impersonation he goes back to his table and starts wetting his inner self again. And we're not talking about bottles of Newcastle Brown Ale here! Oh no, the man was on the most expensive champagne he could get. So what he did, was spending thousands of pounds on ammunition to throw up. What a waste – and this goes for the booze too!

He was a nutter anyway, our Gazza. In his days with Rangers, he once bought a Xmas present for our chairman, mister David Murray. Thick, grey, woollen socks. Very thoughtful, one would say, with those long and cold Scottish winters. Just that Murray didn't have any legs any more. The poor guy spent his days in a wheelchair.

Nevertheless, despite the fact that I never stuck a finger down my throat, the alcohol was getting the better of me. I knew it. At times I couldn't handle it. And I did the stupidest things with a bellyful of booze – to gain respect, which was the biggest irony of all. Being silly, in my opinion, meant being strong. And I had to be strong, as a professional footballer, because if you're weak they slaughter you. Complicated, eh?

I also drank to give my confidence a boost. In the beginning it worked, but later on it turned against me. Problems were piling up. I didn't come home any more, didn't attend training sessions, didn't pay my bills . . . There was this thick fog inside my head.

So, yes, I was more than happy that Peter Kay was going to get me off the booze. At least mostly off the booze, I told myself. Not the full 100 per cent – no way was teetotal the idea. I mean, back home in Glasgow, there would be the occasional pint or two. Okay, I know what the mantra is for AA attendees: 'One is too much, a thousand ain't enough.' But I was convinced I could handle myself after Hampshire. A beer once in a while wouldn't turn me into this monster again, would it?

As I checked in I didn't have a clue as to how things would work in the clinic. Peter had told me some details over the phone, but the information simply hadn't stuck. Not a problem, according to him. He fully understood I was on a different planet. 'Just let things happen' was his advice.

So that's what I did: let things happen. And it all went very smoothly. After a few days of getting to know the place, the therapy really started. I was taken from the main building to a smaller abode further away, almost like a normal home. This, I was told, was to make the patient feel at ease. Still, it felt strange. At Rangers I had been the top dog. Here I was just as important as anyone else – I wasn't important at all. Nobody was.

For the first time in years I found myself in an environment where fame and fortune were totally irrelevant. And I was dealing with it quite well. Because I didn't do too many concessions. I was who I was, and it was for the others to accept it or not.

So, I still tried to crack a joke or two. For instance, there was this guy who was suffering from obsessive tidiness. Everything had to be spotless. He would throw a fit if he noticed something that should've been cleaned. I couldn't stop myself throwing as many breadcrumbs on the floor as possible, just to annoy him. He hated me for it – almost as much as the others did for walking down the corridor in the middle of the night blowing a party horn. Innocent fun, people, honest!

As I wasn't doing any real harm to anybody I wasn't punished for my pranks, but they didn't make me a very popular guest! Not that I could get away with murder though.

One day I asked permission to go to London to buy clothes, as I still only had the football stuff from Johannesburg. 'Back in a few hours!' I claimed. Now, that was a bit too transparent. The therapists sensed that I would go straight to the pub – of which, you know, there are a few in London – so they didn't want to let me go just like that. We came to an agreement: me and a few other patients were allowed to make the journey but only if we were supervised by some of the medical staff.

I agreed. At least I would have a bit of distraction. At least I would miss out on one of those boring counselling sessions. You know, the ones in which you have to talk about yourself and your weaknesses. I hated them. I mean, they weren't exactly like the post-match interviews I was used to giving. The sessions away from the clinic were a particular nuisance. All of a sudden you had to face a bunch of perfect strangers and tell them about your battles with the bottle. Dreadful.

I've always been more of a listener anyway, and one who laughs very easily. The moment one of those professional cricket players in my clinic started talking about his addiction to pot, I simply couldn't stop grinning.

Talking about pot . . . On one of those away sessions, I heard of a housewife's struggle with a special type of pot. A teapot! Well, a kettle, actually. You know, the ones that whistle. And it was the whistling, believe it or not, that had driven her to drinking. Booze, not tea!

Still, I had a lot of respect for these women. Housewives who became addicted after they were widowed really moved me. Their stories hit me right between the eyes, much more than the drivel of so-called movie stars, singers and models, who kept telling everyone how difficult life had become for them. Screw them! If anyone was having a really hard time, it was those lonely widows. Not famous, not rich, just hooked.

Their stories were touching and meant much more to me than those of the entertainment business dropouts. Like one filthy rich model, who once giggled that she had had a relapse over the weekend and admitted taking drugs during, quote, 'one hell of an orgy', unquote! When I heard that shit, I really felt sorry for those poor housewives . . .

When it came to learning how to speak in public, I was a pretty fast learner. What helped was that for the first time my audience didn't include people who detested me. Nobody saw me as the bad egg. They actually thought I was a nice geezer. That, I must say, was a huge relief. And in the end – surprise, surprise! – I even enjoyed those sessions. So when, in the third week, I had to do a public speech about my rather bizarre life, I had a ball. Standing on a chair, chatting about all that had happened, felt great. Mind you, most people there had written their life story down on a simple sheet of paper. One lousy sheet! I had so much to tell that I appeared with a pile of paperwork the size of this book.

As I told them about running naked through the plane, throwing the chairman into the pool and waking up in a pink room not knowing where I was, they were all gazing at me with their mouths wide open. In the end, I was rewarded with hysterical laughter. I felt like a stand-up comedian!

To me, this really felt like therapy. Throwing things out, being honest, not building a wall around me any more: man, I loved the new, vulnerable Fernando! I didn't think about sex any more, nor about alcohol. Didn't have time for it inside the clinic. I was . . .

Hold on! Of course I noticed the odd beautiful woman.

'Open the door – now!' That's what I shouted when we were in London on our much anticipated shopping spree. I was standing on the kerb, waiting for the traffic light, as the silver BMW stopped next to me. Inside the car were three dazzling lasses. As one of them opened the car window I said it again. 'Open the door, so I can jump in!'

It was meant to be funny, to stir things up a bit. But they did open the door. And I, being the gentleman I am, stepped in. 'Now, let's go!'

Peter, my minder for the day, totally freaked out. Especially as the BMW really took off. With Peter running behind it, screaming that the girls should stop, it was like a scene out of a comedy.

Eventually the car did stop. It was just a practical joke, Pete!

The joke may have stopped there, but the entire incident was far from over. When we wandered back to the traffic lights, we noticed that the rest of the group had disappeared. Peter was close to exploding.

After a bit of searching we found them all, and so in the end the entire group returned safely to the fairytale castle where we all lived happily ever after. Oh, and yours truly got a warning, but he's had worse than that in the past.

During my stay at the clinic I did an awful lot of workouts. I didn't train with a ball – there wasn't one to be found – but I kept in shape with running and cycling. I was even eating healthy food. All these efforts to prevent my career fizzling out and I was still only 29!

Okay, my Rangers days were over, no doubt about that, but other clubs might be interested in a strong and healthy Fernando Ricksen. Hence this display of Fighting Spirit.

After a few weeks I was fitter than ever, also thanks to the yoga and shiatsu I was doing. Not always the nicest way of spending an hour, I can tell you. The Japanese body therapy, during which they push their thumbs and fingers into your flesh, is a killer. But I didn't cry! I was 'that hard man from Rangers'.

After leaving the clinic in August, a much better Fernando Ricksen showed his face at, well, Glasgow Rangers. I had to, as I was still on the payroll. Le Guen didn't want to see me on the training pitch with the rest of the squad, so I had to exercise on my own. At eight o'clock every morning. Touching a ball was forbidden. I just had to run, run, run.

This, I'm convinced, was designed to humiliate me. Nevertheless, I did what Le Guen told me to do. I didn't get angry. I didn't sabotage things. I didn't give him any ammo. He was not going to kick me out, oh no. Fat chance, buddy, I'm not giving you the pleasure! If I do what you tell me to do you won't have a reason to fire me.

Barry Ferguson, however, did become one of his victims. After taking the captain's armband off him, the hateful manager sent him away, for whatever reason. At that point I knew it: Le Guen was about to be given his marching orders.

And I was right: on 4 January 2007, only three days after downgrading Barry, Mr Le Guen was shown the way to the nearest Job Centre. That made him the manager with the shortest employment in the history of Glasgow Rangers Football Club.

Now that sums it all up, doesn't it? Okay, it may be easy to say now, after all these years, but looking back I am absolutely certain that Le Guen would have made it in Scotland if he had kept Barry Ferguson and me in the squad. The two of us, pure-blooded warriors, would have kept him in the saddle. It's just that we never got the chance to prove it. Not even after my return from rehab. The man simply ignored me. It struck me as sad and narrow-minded, but I laughed about it. That's me after rehab for you: stronger and more assertive, a lot more positive and a lot less selfish. Just as Peter Kay had promised.

It was just a pity that, without being allowed to kick a ball, a possible new club was now further away than ever. So I was more than surprised when Dick Advocaat called me one day and asked me how I was.

Now, when Dick asks you how things are, he's not just shooting the breeze. He is genuinely interested in, well, how things are. Dick's words always come straight from the heart.

I told him I was all right-ish and ready to battle myself. 'I see what I've done wrong. I've accepted it. Now it's up to me to fight back.'

Now some of you might see Dick as a grumpy little fella. Well, let me tell you one thing: that's wrong. Yes, he's a fanatic when it comes to football and he always wants to win. He is straight and to the point. But at the same time he is the nicest person you can imagine. Dick is honest, unlike most people in professional football. He is unique.

The best moment to see the real Dick – no joke intended here – is when you're having a meal with him in a restaurant. Especially when his wife is there too. Off comes the armour. What's left is a friendly, light-hearted man with a sense of humour.

Some see him as a full-blown money-grabber. I don't. If the man can snatch a few quid – like for instance when he swapped the Belgian Football Association for the Russian one in 2010 – why shouldn't he? Wouldn't you if you had the chance? Maybe he earned some money on my transfers. I never asked him. So what? Does that make him a criminal? Thanks to Dick I have lived in beautiful houses in beautiful cities. Thanks to him I have played for some of the most fantastic clubs in the world, with whom I have won numerous prizes. To me, that is what counts.

We didn't talk about football during that phone call. It was just personal stuff.

A few days later Dick called me again. This time he wanted to know whether I'd be interested to come to Russia. Russia! He had just signed a contract with Zenit, the ambitious club from the wonderful city of Saint Petersburg. His task was to fulfil its ambitions. And, in order to do so, he needed a few tough players. Hard workers. Players like, well, me.

I was surprised. Russia – it didn't sound too attractive to me. I was raised during the Cold War, and all that sprang to mind were images of the old Soviet Union. It was grey there, wasn't it? And people didn't smile.

Dick sensed my hesitation. And out came the tour guide in him. According to Dick, Saint Petersburg was a wonderful city. Life wasn't just good over there, it was fantastic!

'Why don't you give it a try?' he said. 'Just hop over for a few days, so you can see it with your own eyes.'

I had nothing to lose, so I agreed. Only a few days later I found myself in a boat on the river Neva with him, his assistant Cor Pot, my agent Rob Jansen and his right-hand woman Esther Goergen. And I couldn't believe my eyes!

A few hours earlier I'd still had my doubts. Pulkovo Airport was a mess, and on our way in to the city we saw one old Soviet apartment block after the other. I thought to myself, do they really want me to play here? And, hey, if the country is as gorgeous as Dick says it is, how come there are hardly any foreign footballers in the Russian league? No, wait, there was this Dutch-Ghanaian bloke, Quincy Owusu-Abeyie, who was playing for Spartak Moscow, but that was about it at the time. Hence the question: if hardly any players from abroad are coming to Russia, then why on earth should I do it?

Anyway, those doubts disappeared on the gentle waves of the river Neva. Wherever I looked I saw the most beautiful ancient buildings, the most fantastic old churches and the most romantic monumental bridges. As if I were in Paris, or Rome. Or, for that matter, Amsterdam.

Oh, and there were other gems too. I saw them walking on the quays and in the streets. Hundreds of Anna Kournikovas and Maria Sharapovas in short skirts, each and every one showing a dazzling pair of pins.

So I said yes, this is where I'm going to play! 'Just prepare the paperwork,' I said to Rob.

Saint Petersburg . . . what a place to make a fresh new start! Okay, I didn't know anything about Russian football, but that was a minor detail, and two days later, on 14 August, I signed the contract. Being a recovering alcoholic with a shambolic past, I didn't have many demands, so I told Rob I would be all too happy with the same salary as in Scotland.

And indeed he managed to get me on the club's payroll for 1.2 million euros a year, just as with Rangers. A good agent, Rob? A brilliant agent! This time it wasn't 1.2 million gross, but . . . you get it. I was going to earn *more* than in Scotland!

Apart from the money, there was the joy of finally playing again and the pleasure of a life without those horrid British tabloids. Oh, and I wouldn't really miss the Scottish climate either. Nor those crazy end-of-year fixtures. Playing football on Boxing Day, okay, but on the first of January? Madness! Sitting all alone in your hotel room on New Year's Eve waiting for next day's match against Aberdeen. Going to sleep at eleven, because you have to be fit for the confrontation. Festive season, my arse! Well, I guess you catch my drift.

Still, nine days after signing for Zenit Saint Petersburg, I was back at Ibrox. We had to play a friendly against Rangers, as part of a certain deal. I loved being back on the holy turf.

Now, a lot of footballers don't like the idea of playing against their former club. Out of respect, they don't celebrate when they've scored a goal. I don't share those sentiments. Okay, I am a Ranger at heart, now and for ever, but I was looking forward to the match. It was an ideal opportunity to show the world how wrong Le Guen had been.

So, I decided to play as I've always played. Hard! Don't act like a softie, all of a sudden. Just don't kick anybody into a wheelchair. After all, these were all former teammates with whom I shared great memories.

Chris Burke was one of them. Good player, Chris. One of Ibrox's best dribblers – and I'm not talking about the baby variant here. Chris had just returned after a spell off due to a serious injury and he replaced Thomas Buffel after an hour. As soon as he walked up to me, I said to him, 'Now, please don't start dribbling tonight. Just make this a nice game of football, please.'

But stubborn Chris didn't do what I told him and started, you guess it, dribbling. Non-stop. It drove me insane. And, to top everything off, he kicked me.

Now *that* was something he shouldn't have done! A couple of minutes later I whacked him and the ball so hard that they both ended up near the dug-out. He was screaming at the top of his voice, poor Chris. It seemed that I had touched his ankle, the very same ankle that had just been cured. Exit Burke. I think he had been on the pitch for about four minutes.

The 30,000 fans were livid. Not only had I kicked out one of their favourite players, in doing so I had also kicked every single one of them in the gut. They were yelling and cursing at me as if I was the biggest scumbag they'd ever seen. In order to protect me Dick took me off.

The walk to the dressing room was one I'll never forget. The Rangers supporters made it clear that they hated me. Yup, that's football for you: hero to zero in literally one kick. Maybe I would have reacted the same had I been sitting in the stands. On the other hand, this was Fernando Ricksen, the man who takes no prisoners. Didn't they remember? Hadn't they always loved that attitude? Did they really think I would be a different player all of a sudden, now that I was playing against them?

Oh, we slaughtered them too: 4–1, thanks to goals by Ho Lee, Igor Denisov, Aleksandr Kerzhakov and Oleksandr Spivak. To me, this was the ultimate proof that I had made the right decision. This Zenit, with among others the mighty Andrey Arshavin, was a team with possibilities – lots of them.

So I left Glasgow with a big smile on my face.

THIRTEEN

RUSSIA

MY FIRST DAY AS a player for Zenit Saint Petersburg seemed to have landed me in jail.

What? Yup, you read it correctly. My first day as a player for Zenit Saint Petersburg seemed to have landed me in jail. In other words, I was in big trouble again, only a few hours after arriving in Russia. Prison was looming and I was so not looking forward to it! My one night behind Glaswegian bars had been bad enough, but the thought of a *Russian* slammer was freaking me out. I'd seen footage on TV, and it was terrifying.

I was cursing like a sailor. Why the fuck do I always have to end up in this kind of shit? Why does this stuff always happen to me? How on earth is it possible? Why me, why me, why *always* me?

And this time it wasn't even my fault!

My next thought was Dick. My manager. I imagined him finding out about this. He would send me straight home, no doubt about it! And he would be right, as I shouldn't have been out at this ridiculous time of night, just a few hours before my first training session. I should have been in bed, in the Corinthia Nevsky Palace Hotel. Alone.

But I wasn't in bed. Instead, I was somewhere on a ring road outside Saint Petersburg. Or, more to the point, next to it, and facing two coppers.

My heart was doing a John Bonham drum solo. I was so nervous. And angry. That goddamn Andrey Arshavin! Why oh why did he have to climb behind the steering wheel when he was as pissed as a parrot? I'd noticed that he was just as befuddled as his fellow passengers Igor Denisov and Aleksandr Anyokov, so, more to the point, why did *I* get into the car with him? And why did he continue to verbally assault the policemen?

Please, Andrey, behave!

He didn't.

Arshavin, Russia's number one footballer at the time, refused to calm down. He kept on screaming and, to make things worse, started to kick the police car, an old-fashioned Lada.

Here we go again, I thought to myself. Then I turned to Arshavin. 'Please, Andrey, stop it.' No reaction. I got scared. Really scared. 'For Christ's sake, Andrey, stop it!'

My brain was working overtime. What if this incident hit the papers? What if somebody from Zenit had to pick us up from the dungeon? Dick thought I was in bed, having some rest before training. He didn't even know I was out. He would go crazy. The media would bring up my past as an alcoholic. Nobody would believe I hadn't been drinking this time.

In the meantime, Arshavin went on and on, and kicked the police car a few more times, as if he was enjoying it. Then he started shoving one of the policemen. What an idiot!

Then, all of a sudden, the sound of muffled kicks stopped. At last, he's calmed down, I thought. Nope, it was a bluff. Andrey hadn't made his point yet. From that moment on, he got even more aggressive. I could hear it in his voice.

Worse still, he was joined by Aleksandr and Igor, who completed the out-of-tune boy band. I had no idea what the three of them were yelling – I'd only been in Russia for a few hours! – but I knew it wasn't an invitation to a tea party.

Now, this could only lead to a severe retaliation. When it comes to policemen, nobody tolerates this kind of behaviour. We would get nicked for sure, the four of us. Never mind that I was as sober as a newborn baby, I had been in the car – front seat. Maybe they held me responsible for, well, everything. What the hell did I know about the Russian law?

So that was it. The ink on my contract wasn't even dry and I would be on a plane back to Holland again. From Russia with grief. Yeah, I saw the three of them looking at me, with their it's-gonna-be-all-right looks. But that was exactly what worried me.

But guess what? It *was* gonna be all right! Different country, different rules. If you're a famous footballer in Russia you can get away with murder (well, almost). So, instead of arresting us or beating the shit out of us with their truncheons, the cops walked away. They even apologised!

I was puzzled, to say the least. As we drove off, on our way to a strip joint called Maximus, I asked Andrey how the hell . . .

'Fernando, this is Russia,' he said, and laughed his lungs out.

He told me that, in between all his kicking, he'd made a quick phone call to the highest police official in Saint Petersburg. He'd had his number for years, in case of a possible emergency. The top guy happened to be an avid Zenit supporter. Problem solved.

On top of that, the phone call wouldn't even have been necessary had it been a bit brighter that night. If the patrolmen had recognised Arshavin there and then, they would have backed off immediately. In Russia Arshavin was (and still is) a God-like figure. Laws don't apply to him.

He even managed to enter Saint Petersburg's most exclusive nightclub wearing flip flops! It was then that I thought, where the hell have I ended up? But I also knew that this was my kinda place!

My first evening in the city had started in a very relaxed way. Cor Pot, who was staying in the same hotel as me, had invited me to a party which was being held by the Dutch Embassy on a boat. Always good for a bit of networking, Pot said. And he was right, of course. It's always handy to know a few notables from the Netherlands.

It was a pleasant evening and I really enjoyed myself. And I didn't touch a drop of alcohol. I couldn't, as the club doctor, Sergey Pukhov, had given me an injection earlier that day. Drinking a drop of the forbidden stuff would have made me as sick as a dog and given me red spots all over the torso, like the best climber in the Tour de France. 'You're not going to like that,' Pukhov predicted.

The aforementioned injection is illegal in many countries, due to the risks. Not so in Russia. On the contrary, it was quite common to give it to people with a severe alcohol problem. When offered one by the club, I thought it would be very ungrateful to refuse. After all, Zenit had rescued me from my Scottish isolation. It was time to give something back, as you say.

Did I really need it? Well, the fact that I'd had my last pint in South Africa all those weeks ago proved that I wasn't really craving it. On the other hand, it wasn't unlikely either that one day I would fall for the temptation of Miss Vodka. So, I reckoned I'd better kill the passion in advance – with an injection that didn't last one night but, gulp, a whole year!

Pot hadn't had a shot. That was obvious, given the amount of hooch he was enjoying, so when he realised he was inebriated he left the party boat. He said he was off to bed but that I could stay if I wanted: the party wasn't over yet. 'No worries about getting back,' he assured me. 'Any cab driver will know our hotel. Otherwise, give me a call, pal.'

I had a better idea. My Norwegian teammate Erik Hagen had been trying to reach me a few times that evening. As I hadn't answered, he'd sent me a text message. The entire team were having a meal downtown and they would like me to drop by and introduce myself.

Excellent idea! I decided to join them. Cor Pot agreed it would be a good opportunity to team up with the guys, and as we said goodbye he told me he was looking forward to seeing me at training the next morning. And he gave me the smile of a gentleman.

Hagen told me where to find the rest of the lads: in Loge, a Serbian fish restaurant. Top place! I would become a regular there in the months to come. Just as I would frequently visit The Flying Dutchman, a seventeenth-century vessel that hosted wild theme parties with the most stunning models. But I'm saving that for later . . .

A few minutes later I was united with the rest of the squad. And my jaw dropped to the floor when I saw them or, more precisely, the table they were sitting at. It was covered with expensive champagne and whisky bottles – most of them empty. No need to ask where the liquid had ended up: inside the players. What a crazy mob!

Don't forget there was training scheduled for, er, a few hours later.

I sat down and ordered a Coke. It didn't even make me feel uncomfortable, to tell you the truth. It gave me a boost! I felt strong among all these weak pissheads.

I had always been told that the Russians were gruff. Well, not these guys! They made me feel welcome from the very first moment. Arshavin told me this was their true character – and among all the empty bottles, he high-fived me.

Arshavin, Denisov and Anyukov became my buddies, despite the fact that they hardly spoke any English. They did know about my past though. I think they found it quite interesting. After a while, they managed to speak the language a lot better, which was a huge relief, as my Russian lessons sucked. Together with Cor Pot I attended a crash course, but without much success. All those Cyrillic characters drove me up the wall, and I didn't finish the lessons. But it wasn't a big deal, as pretty soon I knew how to speak Russian football lingo – and that was basically all I needed. And off the field, there were always my fellow footballers from the Czech Republic, Croatia, Hungary, Belgium, South Korea and Norway who did know how to make themselves understood in English.

Gradually, more and more Russian players started to speak the language – thanks to Dick. Instead of him learning Russian, he sent them on an English course.

The players didn't object. On the contrary, they loved it! They had two lessons a week, but they fancied the idea of having them each and every day. Eventually the lectures became so popular that Dick had to do something about it.

As it turned out, it wasn't the education itself that the boys loved so much. It was the teacher. An absolute stunner. And they shagged her. One at a time.

When Dick found out he quickly replaced her – probably with an ugly bloke – and all of a sudden going to English class wasn't that popular any more!

Much later on, players like Vladislav Radimov complained about the fact that Dick didn't speak a word of Russian. I thought that was *chush' sobach'ya* – 'bullshit' in Russian. I could fully understand Dick's decision. Russian is a very complex language. You don't learn it just like that; it takes years and years. According to Radimov, Dick couldn't pass on emotions via an interpreter. No emotions? Look at the man's face! Even if he had started to speak Chinese, you would still understand what he meant! It didn't surprise me though that, of all people, it was Radimov who came up with this. He was always against us.

So, back to the fish restaurant, which was now about to close. It was Arshavin – honest! – who came up with the idea of visiting a pole-dancing club. I had to be inaugurated! There was no objection from me, especially after they told me that in Russia, unlike in Great Britain, you were allowed to touch the girls. The thought alone sent a frisson of excitement through my body.

The only thing that worried me was the state my teammates were in. My God, they were drunk! So I suggested we take a taxi. Andrey just laughed. It wasn't going to be a cab, but instead Anyukov's enormous Toyota Land Cruiser. There was enough space for half a football team.

First, I thought they were joking. They could hardly walk – and that included the driver. Oh my God, he would kill himself, and me too!

In the car park I told them that maybe, maybe it wouldn't be a bad idea if Mr Coca-Cola here took the wheel. Yes, it was a bad idea, said Andrey, who climbed into the driver's seat. And then I joined him in the passenger's seat. Wrong, wrong, wrong! But I still did it.

After only 100 metres we heard the sirens . . .

Police! On my first night in Saint Petersburg. Don't tell me I was in trouble already.

'Don't worry,' said Arshavin.

And, as I soon found out, he was right. There was no need to worry. Without any casualties we reached club Maximus, my soon-to-be second home.

That night on the highway was my initiation. It was my first experience of Russia's corruption. 'For sure there's more to come!' Arshavin said with a wink.

One thing I always had to do, they said, was to give the officers some money the moment they stopped you. Bribery, in other words.

'And then, Fernando, everything will be all right.'

Even our team manager Fedor Lunnov gave me similar advice. 'Always have some cash on you, Fernando. Or otherwise a Zenit shirt, or a banner. Policemen like those as well!' But, as Fedor explained, there were certain rules. One: never give the money directly to an officer! 'That's too obvious. Put the cash on their dashboard, so they can take the roubles themselves.'

In order to stay as incognito as possible, I took to driving around Saint Petersburg in a Ford Focus. It was unlikely that a regular car like that would draw any attention. In a Hummer or a Ferrari the coppers would see me coming from miles away, and I didn't want that.

No, it wasn't a good idea to hit the streets of Saint Petersburg in my blood-red Ferrari, like I was used to in Glasgow. I even drove to Rangers matches in it. Exposing my beloved, expensive Ferrari to the Russian traffic was another thing that I didn't fancy, given that most Russians don't even have a driving licence! Yeah, forgeries bought for 300 euros.

Unsurprisingly car crashes were quite common. And people died in those crashes. In March 2011, hours before the UEFA Cup match against FC Twente, Marina Malafeeva, beloved wife of goalkeeper Vyacheslav Malafeev, lost her life. I wasn't playing for Zenit any more, but it still hit me hard. Such a tragedy, she was a mother of two . . . When things like that happen I'm not a hard bastard any more. When the wife of my former teammate Konstantin Zyryanov got so depressed that she jumped off the eighth floor of an apartment block, holding her four-year-old daughter, I got shivers all over. At these times football is the least important thing on earth.

Unfortunately Project Ford Focus didn't work. The cops stopped me constantly. And I didn't even look like a foreigner – I was wearing a furry hat! I'd even adopted the Russian driving style – overtaking left and right, showing no fear at all.

Most of the time I didn't know why they'd stopped me. The very first time, somewhere in town, I hadn't been drinking and I wasn't driving too fast, so what was going on? That was my question to them too.

As the conversation was leading nowhere – they didn't speak English, I didn't speak Russian – I decided to call our team manager Fedor. 'Call me if you get in to trouble, Fernando. No matter what time of day or night,' he'd told me.

He picked up the phone immediately.

'Fedor,' I said, 'I think I've got a problem.'

Silly Fernando had a problem indeed, as he had been stupid enough to give them his passport and driving licence. And they refused to give the documents back.

Fedor kept his cool. 'Just let me talk to the guys, okay?'

Without asking any questions, I pushed my cell phone against the ear of one of the representatives of the strong arm of the law. Twenty seconds later I got it back. We then knew the accusation: I had been speeding. According to them.

'Just pay, Fernando. Even if you are innocent. Pay and they'll let you go.'

I did object to this, but only internally. I didn't want any hassle, but it was ridiculous, as I'd been driving at twelve miles an hour.

Next question: how much to pay? I didn't have the slightest idea. And Fedor had hung up. I didn't want to insult them with my donation, as they'd come after me again. How about, let's see, 1,000 roubles? That's about £17, and quite a lot of money for the average Russian. So I grabbed a 1,000-rouble note and laid it on their dashboard, just as Fedor had advised.

It was enough. I got my valuables back and was allowed to continue my journey.

Now, this used to happen once or twice a week. Each week! And they had one daft story after the other. Crossing a line was one of them; neglecting a red traffic light another; speeding was the most popular one.

Still, I continued driving by myself. I didn't want a chauffeur from the club, like Dick and Cor had, because that would limit my freedom. With my own car I could go wherever I wanted. If I could find 'wherever', that is, as the signs were all in Cyrillic, so I used to miss the odd turn-off. I often ended up in the outskirts, and they weren't the nicest (or safest!) places to drive around for two hours, I can assure you. Finding a local who spoke English was practically impossible. But, hey, it was another adventure!

After a while, I felt some sympathy for those cops – or at least some understanding. Russia is ostensibly a rich country, but there is a lot of poverty too. Policemen only earn a pittance a month, not enough to survive on in an expensive city like Saint Petersburg. Unemployment benefits don't exist in Russia, so being on the dole isn't an alternative. They simply have to lay their hands on that extra bit of highway cash to make it to the end of the month. And that was why you had to be extra careful during the festive season – that time of year when families really need some extra pocket money.

Also, once you'd paid them, it was over and done with. No endless red tape, as in Holland, which can lead to fines and court if you forget to pay them.

Corruption was everywhere. Want your driving licence? Wait for two months. Unless, like one of my female friends did, you give a public servant some cash and suddenly you're a priority.

So, I soon picked up that this was the way to deal with things. I've no idea how much money I spent that way, but it must have been a lot. The advantage was that nobody bothered me any more. And when they found out I was this famous footballer from Zenit

– albeit not one as popular as Arshavin – I hardly got busted at all.

And fraud within football itself? I can't prove anything, but I do have my doubts. Take, for instance, Vladislav Radimov in the match against Rubin Kazan, October 2006. He handed the ball to an opponent, so he could score easily. And this didn't happen once, not even twice, but three bloody times in a row! Now, I can't say it stank, but it certainly smelled odd . . .

Match fixing? I made that connection a few years later, as the phenomenon became popular. Once again, I can't prove anything, but it still frustrates me. Thanks to that suspicious 0–3 against Rubin Kazan, our chances to win the title disappeared like snow in the Sahara. We ended up in a disappointing fourth place.

And this wasn't an isolated incident. Two weeks later, when we had to face main rivals and later champions CSKA Moscow, strange things happened again. Once again, as in the confrontation with Rubin Kazan, we were the better of the two teams. But we lost.

It was a shambles. Handball in the goal, after Arshavin was about to score. Two incorrect offside decisions against Andrey. A penalty after their centre-forward, Vágner Love, fell over the ball, with none of us near him. Daniel Carvalho, their Brazilian midfielder, scored from the dot, and red-faced Dick was jumping around as if he were on fire. He continued to do so, way after the final whistle had faded.

Shortly after, the referee was suspended – a wise decision from the Russian FA. But it was useless for us – we didn't get a rematch. It gave me the impression that everything was allowed in the ongoing battle between Russia's biggest cities, Moscow and Saint Petersburg.

It was always a high-voltage encounter when we met CSKA. Okay, it wasn't as much of a madhouse as the Old Firm, but, still, the confrontations with the club from the capital were rather unpleasant. They found us, the new kids on the block, a nuisance. For years and years they had been untouchable, and all of a sudden there were these rascals from up north trying to steal their crown. They did everything to prevent us from being the country's best – and I had great difficulties with that.

And there was more I had to get used to; the fact that simple things almost always turned into complex things. Like, for instance, dealing with things such as a bank account. I didn't have one in the beginning, but – surprise! – I was in need of some cash. So I called Zenit and asked them to transfer some to my old Citibank account.

'No problem,' they said. 'Just come to our office downtown. That's where our safe is. We make sure there will be some money for you once you arrive.'

The aforementioned money was part of my salary. With it, they told me, I could go to any bank and open an account, just like that.

I was in a very good mood when I drove to the office, the next day, but once I'd entered the place I thought they were taking the piss. You know the kind of plastic bags you get at Tesco, or any supermarket? Well, there were two of them, and they weren't filled with groceries. The two bags were *loaded* with money! Total amount: 3.5 million roubles (£80,000)!

'Here you are,' the clerk said, as he handed me the bags. As if they were filled with old newspapers.

But . . . hang on, what was I supposed to do with this? Go out for a walk, whistling? 'Hey, what are you staring at? Never seen a guy with two shopping bags full of money?' In Russia, they'd kill you for a tenth of that sum.

'What's the problem?' the clerk asked. 'You wanted some cash, didn't you?' He noticed the fear in my eyes. 'Don't worry, son. Nothing will happen to you.'

And he meant it. So out I went, shaking like a turkey around Christmas, to my car. The heaviest few metres of my life – literally, as the weight of the bags was enormous, because they were filled with 1,000-rouble notes.

During my drive to the Citibank, on the other side of town, I was praying that the cops wouldn't stop me. Not this time. Please, not this time. 'No, officer, I haven't robbed a bank.'

I reached the bank, but, shit, no parking spot! Wait, there was one a few hundred metres away, but no way was I going to take the risk again. I parked the Ford Focus on the pavement, right in front of the entrance. Big deal if they fined me; it would be cheaper than getting mugged. And how long was it going to take, anyway? Hand over the money, open an account . . . piece of cake, surely.

So in I walked. 'Good afternoon, I am a professional player from Zenit and I would like to open an account. Oh, and I would like to put this in it.'

The man behind the desk looked at me as if I was a complete lunatic. 'Not possible, sir.'

'Not possible? What do you mean "not possible"?'

'You are a foreigner, so you should have asked for this in advance. Procedure, sir.'

I got angry. Started to call him names. 'I'm not leaving the place!' and 'Look how much money this is! They'll murder me on the street!'

The man consulted his superior. Then it was, 'Okay, just this once . . . but we have to count it. Three times. Procedure, sir.'

Now try to picture the scene: a slow bank employee counting a mountain of bank notes – three times. After two hours of waiting I'd had enough. 'It's fine, I believe you,' I tried to tell him. 'There's no need to count it for a third time.'

The employee shook his head. He really had to count the notes one, two, three times. 'Procedure.' And after that . . . *a fourth time, with the machine!* Just to be sure, you know.

Three hours later I had my bank account. And it was loaded. More good news: my Ford Focus was still on the pavement, and its flashlights were still on. Plus, I didn't even have a fine! A day well spent, after all.

Anyway, time for a flashback to that first night in Saint Petersburg. Remember the strip joint I'd entered with my drunk buddies Arshavin, Denisov and Anyukov? Guess who was there, lying in a chair, plastered . . . Cor Pot.

Yup, the assistant who had been so 'tired' that he had to go 'to bed'. Somewhere along the line he must have changed his mind. Anyway, he was completely wasted, so in the end I had to take him back to the hotel and put him to bed. That's Cor for you, a man who likes to party.

Unlike Dick. He hardly left his super-duper suite on the top floor of the Kempinsky Hotel. It was a wonderful room with a breathtaking view over the city and its famous museum, the Hermitage, but I wonder if Dick ever noticed the beauty of it. All the Little General did was watch DVD footage of our future opponents, for hours and hours and hours. But, he was as prepared as a human being can be.

Only after finishing all his homework was there time for relaxation. In Dick's case this meant switching to satellite television and watching . . . *more* football! Sometimes until two in the morning.

Cor, as you may have guessed, was a totally different person. After watching a DVD once, he thought that was enough. Time to go out. Time to have a bite to eat with Fernando – preferably at club Maximus. An amazing place with delights wherever you looked: on your plate and on the poles.

Yeah, it wasn't a bad choice after all, Mother Russia!

FOURTEEN

A NEW HOME

I WAS CONSTANTLY SURPRISED at the things that were happening to me in Russia. And we're talking about my *second* day in Saint Petersburg here!

It was the morning of our first training session at the ground in Udelnaya, a neighbourhood as grey as Arsene Wenger's hair after a string of defeats with Arsenal. I was in top shape. Of course I was; I hadn't been drinking the night before. No headache. No hangover. Perfect. I hadn't slept that much, obviously, but I wasn't tired. To be honest, I'm rarely tired, and can function on just a couple of hours' sleep a night.

The other guys had a lot more problems. My God, it was like I'd been transferred to Comedy Capers FC! I was expecting Laurel and Hardy any moment.

Arshavin was there, but at the same time he wasn't. He was still pissed and, because of the state he was in, Russia's best footballer managed to . . . fall over the ball! At first I thought he was joking. But he wasn't. He simply couldn't stand up straight! And he wasn't the only one . . .

It was ten a.m.

Dick saw it too. I was wondering how long it would take him to put his foot down. Not long. A few more half-baked somersaults later, and he started kicking some balls (leather ones, don't get me

165

wrong!) before he took off, gesticulating wildly. The man was not amused!

We didn't see him again that morning. I didn't even get the chance to tell him how happy I was to be one of the boys again, after all those weeks.

When Dick's away the boys will play, and that's exactly what we did: playing a little game of footy without a referee. It was the only option. There simply wasn't anybody left who could blow the whistle, as Cor had taken off too. Not that he went immediately.

'Cor?'

'Cor!'

'Cor!'

'Cor, are you coming with me or what?'

Poor Cor was oblivious. And it wasn't on purpose. He was still a bit intoxicated himself after me dragging him out of club Maximus and putting him to bed. No doubt Dick wasn't aware of that!

Strangely enough, after this farcical gathering which was meant to be a professional training session, I thought, I'm gonna have one hell of a time playing with these guys. Together we're gonna win the title. I know it!

Out of the 24 players on the pitch, 20 had been drinking the night before. It was unheard of – and this comes from a guy who has played in Scotland! But, these lads were a single unit. A unit of Fighting Spirits.

They were all international players representing their respective countries. There were the Russians, of course, including Andrey Arshavin, Igor Denisov, Vyacheslav Malafeev and Aleksandr Anyukov, later to be joined by fellow countrymen Pavel Pogrebnyak, Igor Semshov, Roman Shikorov, Oleksandr Horshkov and Konstantin Zyryanov. Then we had South Korean Young-Min Hyun, as well as Martin Skrtel from Slovakia, Ivica Krizanac from Croatia, Radek Sirl from the Czech Republic and Anatoliy Tymoshchuk, the cannonball from Ukraine.

Yes, unknown names to most of you, I'm sure, but, believe me, these guys knew how to play a game of football! Especially Anatoliy, our new captain. Dick called him 'the best libero in the world'. Later on, he would win the Champions League with Bayern Munich. You can't do that if you're a total flapjack!

Yes, there were all sorts and in all conditions, in this squad. But birds of a different feather can still flock together, as we proved. And when, on top of that, the training sessions are good, prizes are up for grabs.

And the training was good! The craftsmanship of Dick and Cor was unsurpassed. I loved the fact that they let us practise with the ball for most of the time, unlike the endless running sessions that were common in Russia.

But Dick wanted high standards – and a lot of the guys had difficulties with that. They were used to Czech coach Vlastimil Petrzela, who did an impersonation of the Invisible Man for most of the time (the players saw him only once a week, on a Friday morning).

With Dick it was a completely different story! He was on the training field every single day. That's how fanatical the wee man is. Only the day after the match before, he let Cor Pot and Russian assistant Nikolai Vorobjev do the training. Dick wanted perfection, full stop, but the players were allowed to laugh – and that was a novelty too. They were even allowed to talk to each other! Unheard of, up until then. Before Dick they had been drilled like robots.

Another thing Dick introduced was giving each other a compliment once in a while. Applaud after a good performance. Simple things, I agree, but they made a difference. Through it, players were creating a tight bond with each other.

Sometimes Dick got angry. And if Dick gets angry . . . Well, ask Arshavin. God in boots in Russia, but Dick didn't spare him. Nobody would normally dare to do a thing like this, but Dick even suspended him in the middle of the season! But, I have to say, Andrey had asked for it . . .

One night before a clash with Spartak Moscow, Arshavin had gone into town, although he wasn't allowed to. Together with Denisov and Anyukov, they cleansed themselves with vodka. Dick erupted when he found out. He felt hurt; he'd thought he could trust his boys. So, he decided they had to be punished – not with a fine, as the guys were loaded, but by putting them on the bench during one of the biggest games of the season.

Russia was astonished, but Dick wasn't impressed. Discipline is discipline, and trust is trust. Dick showed the lads who the real hot shot was: not three Russian superstars, but a guy from the streets of The Hague. And it wasn't until the trio apologised, on Zenit's website, that Dick put them back in his squad. They learned their lesson well!

Being the little nosy parker he is, Dick clashed with more people than just his players. On certain days, he even felt the urge to shout at Cor. As he let rip in Dutch, I could understand every single word of it. It was highly amusing; still, Dick and Cor agreed on nine out of ten things, so their verbal fights were rare.

Cor had a thick skin, so he could deal with Dick's displays of unhappiness quite well. Fedor Lunnov couldn't. After having had the easiest job in Russian football for years, all of a sudden he had to accept the fact that Big Brother, sorry, Little General was watching him – every single day. If Fedor did something that Dick didn't approve of, he could expect the worse.

According to Dick, Fedor didn't do anything right. Socks? Wrong. Training shoes? Wrong. Tickets? Wrong. I felt sorry for Fedor, as he was constantly on the receiving end of Dick's wrath. But what could he do? Nothing! And he knew it. If Dick wanted something to happen, it had to happen. No question. I'd heard stories of chairmen or club owners who entered the dressing room with a view on who was going to play and who wasn't. Not so at Zenit. Sergey Fursenko, our president who had arrived from mighty sponsor Gazprom, never showed up amidst the smelly socks and sweaty shirts. Rightly so, as Dick wouldn't have tolerated that. He would have thrown him out, for sure.

He'd done that with Sean Connery already! Shortly before a Rangers match, chairman David Murray thought it would be a nice idea to introduce the one and only James Bond to us. The Little General didn't agree and sent him away.

The name is Advocaat, Dick Advocaat.

Dick ruled at Zenit. He decided everything. If the pitch wasn't to his liking, Gazprom gave him new grass. Just like that. It made sense. A good pitch would improve the football and lead to results. And good results were what Zenit wanted from him. It was as simple as that.

Although not quite Michel Roux Jr, Dick even took care of the food. In the Ritz-Carlton, our regular hotel in Moscow, he would discuss the menu with the chefs. It had to be proper athletes' fare, not just pub grub.

Next step: private hotel rooms for everybody. Just as I was used to with the Dutch national team. The Zenit players were grateful for this. Sometimes, in places outside Moscow, hotels weren't big enough to give every player his own room. Take Grozny, for instance. Horrid place. I've been in, well, thousands of hotel rooms, but this one in the capital of Chechnya was the worst of the lot. It had a star – yes, one! – but even that was overrated. No restaurant, no internet, nothing! Actually, we couldn't find a decent eating place in the whole of Grozny, so we ended up having dinner at . . . an old lady's down the road!

There we were, a bunch of spoiled-rotten footballing millionaires, waiting for this Grozny granny to serve us whatever she had cooked; at her kitchen table, in the slum that she called home. Top football in Russia . . .

She did her best, this old woman, but the food was – how to say this without being rude to her? – well, strange, and it stank! It looked (and smelled) like a pile of zombie body parts after a car crash. Yuck! It was impossible to eat it without heaving it back up involuntarily.

From then on, I always made sure I had some cookies and candy bars with me. If possible, I would have taken my own bed as well. Pigs would have demanded another one too, in that 'one star' hotel in Grozny, which was hardly more than a shed. So, when I heard the news that Ruud Gullit was going to be the new manager at Terek Grozny, I was puzzled, to say the least. I thought the former Rasta

Man had lost it! Not because Ramzan Kadyrov, the club's suspicious chairman, paid him with bribe money. I didn't want any of that. C'mon, whoever objects to that is simply envious. Did this make Ruud a criminal? Had he killed anyone? Please! Some people have all the luck; others don't have any. That's life!

I was thinking more about the practical side of his decision. What was he going to do there? After years of war Grozny was reduced to nothing. So Gulliman must have lived somewhere else. Like the players of Guus Hiddink's FC Anzhi, who didn't stay in the too-dangerous Daghestan, but in Moscow.

Incidentally Gullit was fired after six months, for spending 'too much time in Grozny's nightclubs'. Nightclubs? What nightclubs? I've only seen soldiers there. They'd stop our bus every five minutes. Checkpoints galore! Unnecessary, I thought initially, until I heard that one week earlier, on the eve of the Grozny v. Kazan match, the Russian army had found a bomb dangling on the door knob of . . . the hotel where we were staying! So the presence of the army *did* make sense!

We were distracted, to put it mildly, but we won the game against Terek Grozny 4–1. That's how professional we were. I didn't feel scared with all those soldiers and tanks around. After all, they weren't going to kill an entire football team, were they? But I was still delighted when the journey home approached. Back to safe and beautiful Saint Petersburg. I don't like places where you hardly see a woman. I'm glad Dick agreed and made our obligatory trips to Grozny as short as possible.

Moscow was the other end of the spectrum. A wonderful city, I loved being there! We always stayed at the Ritz-Carlton, a stone's throw away from Red Square. Now, I'm not the world's most cultural person, but I've always found it a fascinating place. HQ of the Russian Federation – impressive! Sitting there, after dinner, with a cup of coffee, enjoying the view of the Kremlin – brilliant!

Sometimes we visited Lenin's mausoleum, which really is beyond imagination. *Enormous*. It was as good as Mao's grave, which I'd seen during my trip to China in 1993, with Fortuna. So, apart from winning the odd Cup, I can say I've seen two of the world's most famous tombs!

Walking through the streets of Moscow was done in my Zenit outfit. No problem at all. Nobody bothered me. The only people who came up to me were Scots who wanted to have their picture taken with me. And they included Celtic fans, which, I must say, made me very proud.

Dick didn't mind that we were wandering around town, as long as we were back in our rooms by eleven. He checked. No problem – we were always in on time.

With girls . . . that was our little secret.

Dick didn't know that. He never saw us leaving the lobby with a lady. Of course not, she had her own key! We would leave it in an envelope at reception. Lots of times, as Dick and I were chatting in the hotel lobby over a last cup of coffee, I would hear the sound of high heels trotting towards the elevator. Got him! And her, later on.

Dick always wanted to be the man in charge, and if things were not going his way he would become abusive, with players, officials, anyone.

And I wasn't an exception. As much as he liked me he could still get very, very angry with me. Like, for instance, on that night in Marbella, January 2007. He was *totally* fed up with me.

'I don't want to see you at Zenit any more. Go and find yourself another club!'

That's the adrenaline, I thought. In a few hours' time he'll have calmed down.

Yes, he calmed down, eventually, but he hadn't changed his mind. 'Sorry, Fernando, your Zenit days are over.'

This was six months after I'd arrived. He told me he'd warned me enough. So there I was, in my hotel room, calling my agent Rob Jansen. 'Rob, we seriously have to search for another club.'

'What have you done *this time*?' he sighed.

I told him that I had fought with Vladislav Radimov during a friendly in Málaga against a local amateur team. I hadn't KO'd him, but it was a punch Mike Tyson wouldn't be too ashamed of.

'Radimov?' Rob asked. 'Your teammate?'

'Yeah,' I answered. 'That's what makes this whole case so, er, complicated.'

No regrets there. The guy had asked for it. I don't tolerate it when an older player curses at youngsters non-stop. Okay, they have to learn things the hard way. After all, so did I. But it has to be done in a reasonable manner. And, more than that, you should be an example to them. Radimov wasn't. He was lazy that game, lazy as hell. And that irritated me, until I couldn't take it any longer.

'For once, keep your big mouth shut!' I yelled at him. 'And if you can't, try saying those things to me, not to the kids!' And I reminded him about his stupid behaviour a few months earlier, which had cost us the title.

Out of respect to him, I'd never broached the subject before. But now I had lost my patience with him. It was time to tell him the truth.

He looked at me sheepishly. This made me even angrier. 'You know what? You're just a lousy footballer! Totally useless! Time to find another job, you talentless jerk!'

I don't know if he heard me. What I do know is that he felt the jab that came with it. Actually, it was more than one blow: it was three. I think. In all honesty, I lost count. He was lucky that Erik Hagen and some other guys stepped in, otherwise I would have finished him.

I'd never been that angry before. And I couldn't calm down. Even after we had been sent off, I still wanted to attack him, but too many teammates were keeping me away from him.

In the dressing room I came to my senses.

The fight was the talk of the town and footage of it was shown all over Spain. No, all over the world! Fighting teammates, that was unique. Big hit on YouTube.

I never liked the guy – he was always badmouthing Dick and me – so it wasn't our first clash. A few months earlier, during a game against FK Rostov, we ended up face to face. Same reason. I think it was poor Martin Skrtel, later of Liverpool fame, who he was trying to humiliate.

Luckily, a day after the Battle of Málaga, Dick told me I could stay. He'd had a meeting with the squad in which the boys told him that they wanted to keep me. They needed a Fighting Spirit in the race to the first title in ages, and there was only a small fine for Radimov and me in the end.

So I was back on the phone to Rob Jansen. He told me he was relieved that Dick had changed his mind, because it had been impossible for him to find me another club. The press had branded me the bad boy again and no team was interested in me any more.

Because of the incident I rose in Zenit's hierarchy. People listened more to me than before. I wonder why . . . No, I don't.

I even came to terms with Radimov. We would never be friends, but 'good colleagues' was a possibility.

We had been in Spain because of the climate. The Russian winter was simply too cold to play football; that's why teams escaped to sunnier places. And not for a few days, like Dutch teams do in winter, but for a few weeks.

Money didn't matter, thanks to our rich sponsor Gazprom. Our training ground in Udelnaya alone, my God! I was used to a locker for my valuables. Unheard of at Zenit – they provided you with an entire room with your own television set! Everybody got dressed and undressed in their private room – very unusual.

And Zenit was ahead of the rest when it came to the medical side of the business too.

I'd noticed that, the day before games, one player after the other would visit our doctor. I was curious. So I decided to do it too. Well, I had a look around the corner and then backed off.

Needles and syringes all over the place. Players hooked up to drips, laughing. It looked like a secret laboratory. I was flabbergasted.

From behind his desk Doctor Pukhov saw me staring. He smiled. 'Want some too?'

He told me they were vitamins. Liquid preparations. According to him, it was magic. 'Makes you recuperate a lot faster. Fit to play another game within a day!'

'Okay, whatever,' I said, not overly enthusiastic.

Without thinking about the possible consequences, I laid down on a bed. In went the needle and I closed my eyes. Not because of the pain, but more out of fear. It was strange! I didn't have a clue what Doctor Pukhov was putting in me. He'd talked to me before he prepared the vaccination, but it was all medical lecture and Russian chit-chat.

As I walked back to my room I was annoyed that I hadn't paid more attention. Okay, it hadn't been blood, but what was this 'liquid energy' that he had given me? All I knew about were vitamin pills, shakes and creatine. But this, this was something I'd never come across before.

I wasn't too happy about it. I kept thinking about Frank de Boer, Edgar Davids and Jaap Stam, who had been caught for the alleged use of nandrolone (an anabolic steroid), way back in 2001. They'd always denied it, but they had been fined nonetheless. I was scared this would happen to me too.

Still, I couldn't imagine Dick taking the risk. Not now, on the verge of Zenit's international breakthrough. He would never allow his players to use dope.

Apart from that, it was no use crying over spilt milk, as the milk was already inside my veins. No way back now. But, man, it worked! I got an energy boost which was beyond imagination. Normally it took me 48 hours to fully recuperate, now I was fit again immediately, ready to play another three games! That came in handy, as we did have to play three games that week.

I liked it so much that I asked for it again. And again and again and again. In the end I was on four fixes a week. After every training session I walked into Pukhov's medical room, where I spent half an hour on the drip. I loved it. It was good for flu too. One shot and I felt like I was in a sauna, sweating it all out. Magic!

Nobody ever tested positive, so I was convinced that it wasn't something illegal. Pukhov, I kept telling myself, must know the boundaries. After all, the man had been the official doctor of the Russian Olympic team. Nevertheless, my fellow teammates hated those doping tests, for the simple reason that they wanted to get away as fast as possible after the match. There wasn't such a thing as a players' lounge, so fun had to be found elsewhere.

I liked the doping tests when I was at Rangers. No, I loved them! You see, in order to make you pee, they provided cans of beer. Drinking beer tickles your bladder, as we all know, and a lot faster than water does. So I took the opportunity to down a few.

Actually, not just a few . . . I made a party out of it, especially when my booze brother Steven Thompson had to submit his urine too. Sometimes we kept drinking until we were completely plastered. And even then I pretended not to be able to piss! I'd swallow another six or seven cans before I could do the trick. Difficult, I can tell you. Hardly capable of standing upright and knowing there's an inspector breathing down your neck – there are easier ways of seeing a man about a dog.

And all the time there was a coach load of players waiting to go back to the hotel. Sometimes they had to wait a full hour before that Ricksen bastard appeared. I didn't care. When I was on the bus, I'd fall asleep.

So, back to Zenit and the supplements. I've always wondered why Dutch and British clubs never used the same methods as Doctor Pukhov. I mean, could the stuff have been illegal, seeing as we could import it anywhere we went, in the UEFA and Champions League tournaments? His hotel bed was quite a sight. I counted at least sixteen syringes on it every time. Only one or two foreign players didn't feel the need. Their choice, but the supplements worked for me! From the first moment on the pitch I was sharp as, well, a needle. Without it, it would take me at least half an hour to get into the game. It also felt as if the last match I'd played was over a week ago. In reality, it was only a matter of days.

All this was part of Gazprom's plans for Zenit Saint Petersburg. Since they had bought 51 per cent of the shares (for 27.9 million euros in 2005), the sky was the limit. No, not even that, as they chartered us our own plane! It was a Boeing, which from the outside looked like an ordinary BA aircraft; the difference was the luxury on board, with fantastic leather seats and, with just us on board, plenty of leg room.

Quite a contrast to my AZ days, when the biggest domestic adventure was a bus drive from Alkmaar to Kerkrade (check your atlas).

Extra bonus: we no longer had to be crammed into a Tupolev, which, as we all know, isn't one of the most reliable aeroplanes in the world.

Not that I was particularly scared of them; most of the time I was asleep. Only once, when the pilot wanted to land in Rostov upon Don, in the southwest of the country, did I get worried. The wind was so strong the guy couldn't keep the aeroplane straight. I was expecting a wing to hit the ground any minute, but it didn't happen, and in the end we landed safely. By the time I was waiting at the conveyor belt I'd forgotten about the incident.

My motto had always been: if we fall down, we fall down. Yeah, simple as that. But I was the only one who thought like that. Most of my mates were terrified of those flying coffins, especially when yet another one fell from the sky, which happened on a fairly regular basis.

Hats off to those pilots, by the way, as some of the landing strips were pretty crappy. Not in Moscow; in the small rural places like Nalchik, Amkar or Tomsk in Siberia. For some reason I always thought their strips wouldn't be able to handle such a big plane as ours.

But, hey, how else were we going to get to an away game? By moped? We're talking about Russia, friends! And Saint Petersburg is way up in the north, somewhere between Finland and Estonia. All our away games, minus the six in Moscow, had to be flown to. Like the ones against FC Luch-Energia in bloody Vladivostok. That's as far southeast as you can get; on the border with China and North Korea! That means a *nine-and-a-half-hour* flight! That's like Glasgow to Jamaica. For a league match!

Due to the length of the trip, lots of clubs lost their away games in Vladivostok. Saint Petersburg was one of them. Until Dick arrived. His secret? He kept our time over there as short as possible, so we could focus on the game and only the game itself. No acclimatising:

we arrived, went to the hotel for a nap, had a bite to eat, drove to the stadium, played the game and took off again that same evening. Therefore we stayed in our normal, everyday rhythm.

Yes, this was hard going, but at the same time I was having the time of my life. I was visiting places I'd never heard of before: Krasnodar, Samara, Yaroslavl, Khimki . . . Or I would go to cities that were totally unappealing to me, like Vladivostok and Grozny. In moments like that, you realise how little you know of this big, wide world. The aforementioned cities are home to millions and millions of people.

Money didn't matter at Zenit. Just look at the transfers. In the summer of 2008 Zenit paid over 30 million euros for a Portuguese midfielder by the name of Danny. They bought him from Dynamo Moscow. It was the highest transfer sum in the history of Russian football. To me, it was further proof of Gazprom's big ambitions.

So I wasn't remotely surprised when, four years later, they spent 80 million Euros in a week, with the purchase of the Brazilian Hulk (yup, that's his real name) and the Belgian Axel Witsel, whose respective clubs were FC Porto and Benfica. However, I was surprised that those guys chose a city like Saint Petersburg – and not just because Russia is much colder than Portugal.

Don't get me wrong. Saint Petersburg is a fantastic place, with an almost American-style 24/7 economy. Bars, restaurants, shops, nightclubs, museums: Saint Petersburg has it all. Even beaches! I used to go water-skiing around Ploshad Lenina, in the northwest. Or I'd hire a boat and sail off to Finland. In summer the place felt like paradise. Add to this the famous White Nights in summer, when the sun hardly goes down, and you get the picture.

Er, did I say White Nights? Yes, I did. And it sounds like White Knights, of which Saint Petersburg has a few. A lot, actually. Racists. Skinheads. Thugs who beat you into a pulp because they don't like the colour of your skin. It's one of Saint Petersburg's biggest problems. Once in a while you'd hear a story about an African guy being violently assaulted in one of the city's outskirts. Terrible, terrible.

Given the fact that lots of Russians are racist, it didn't surprise me when the Zenit ultras came up with a flyer in which they said they wouldn't tolerate black and/or homosexual players within their club. The 'request' was firmly rejected.

Raised by communist parents, those guys are as patriotic as hell. It will take them years and years until they think the way we do in Western Europe. What I did find strange, however, was their hunt for gay players. Because they didn't exist. At least, not on the surface. Not a single bloke in Russian football has come out of the closet, but statistically speaking, they must be there. Not that I ever suspected anyone in all my years there.

Professional football is not a safe sport to be in as an openly gay guy. You'd be slaughtered! Unlike in swimming, speed skating or horse racing, homosexuality is still a big taboo in soccer. I can understand it, to tell you the truth. A bisexual footballer? At least he shags women half of the time. As a professional footballer you enjoy a high status when you can say that you've bedded loads of women. But a totally gay man? He'd have a hard time in the dressing room – no joke intended. Seriously, it's sad, but a gay player simply won't make it in football. It's a macho world – and not just in Russia.

But back to the racist thugs. Was it really a coincidence that I never had a black teammate during my stay at Zenit? Don't think so! It would've been a hostile environment for well-respected colleagues like Jimmy Hasselbaink and Mario Melchiot. Multicultural Moscow, okay, but conservative Saint Petersburg, no. It was even worse: the fans wanted a 100 per cent Russian squad, in fact 100 per cent local squad – preferably without boys who had ever played for a team in Moscow! Typical.

And they were loud. My God, those supporters were loud! Louder even than the Scots. And it wasn't just to support the team; it was a display of rebellion against law and order. That's why the surroundings of the stadium looked like a war zone on match days.

It mainly kicked off when we played against Spartak Moscow. A lot of blood was spilt on those days. People even got killed. Once, at a Cup match a mere ten years ago, no less than twelve Zenit supporters lost their lives. Since then, it's always been chaotic when the two meet. For instance, in Moscow, in 2008, *700* people got arrested!

Fortunately I've never been a target for the Zenit ultras. They saw me as one of them: somebody who was prepared to fight for the club, and not just some overpaid foreigner who only came to collect the cash. They cheered when I kicked an opponent, recognised my Fighting Spirit, and saw me for the tattooed hunter that I am.

And I loved it!

FIFTEEN

SUCCESS

YES, I ENJOYED SAINT Petersburg more and more. And I was performing well, despite the extremely high speed the Russians played at. Had to gasp for a bit of oxygen now and again, but that wasn't so unusual. After all, I had a six-month hiatus behind me, in terms of playing top-level football. I even started to score, from the right midfield position, as the goalkeepers from FK Rostov and Spartak Nalchik found out.

I was back!

My progress didn't go unnoticed and soon I was offered a new contract. By the end of November, less than three months after my arrival, they changed my status from 'hired' to 'bought'. They really believed in me.

I signed until the end of 2010, didn't think twice about that. As I said, I loved life in Saint Petersburg and I was away from the prying eyes of the press. You know, Russian reporters knew a thing or two about me too, but at least they had the decency to keep it to themselves. Like that ring-road incident on my first night, for instance, which definitely would have made the Scottish headlines had it happened in Glasgow. Not so in Russia. Here, they only wrote about how a footballer played his game of football. They simply weren't interested in the things we did before or after the match. Or, they weren't *allowed* to write about those things. It wasn't unthinkable: a multinational like Gazprom is quite powerful. But what about freedom of the press, I can hear you say. But, to me, it was nice as it was. I wanted to stay here as long as possible.

So, no paparazzi, no tabloids; Fernando could very happily could go into town. Which, of course, he did – a lot. Staying at home I would miss out on the sight of all those women, who were so much more beautiful than anywhere else in the world. Not a single one of those stunners wore jeans. They all had skirts on – short ones. Below that, a pair of dazzling pins with heels the height of a skyscraper. Those chicks walk around as if they are on a catwalk – day in, day out, night in, night out. Russian women visit their hairdresser, pedicure, beauty salon and gym on an almost daily basis. And, boy, they know how to flirt!

And they do it with every single bloke, not just with the rich and famous. You've got to have the radar for it. I do. But when I had a Dutch TV crew around me, I really had to point it out to them.

I liked the fact that those TV guys dropped by. Okay, they were in town to shoot an item about Russians and HIV, and I was just an extra item, but I still enjoyed it. It was nice to welcome the occasional Dutch journalist. They didn't visit me that often, you know. Typically Dutch: things were going fine, so I wasn't interesting to the public. But after something negative, like that fireworks thing in Scotland, I would be all over the pages. Mind you, back home nobody knew that I was voted Scottish Footballer of the Year!

There was a crew from the Dutch arm of MTV, and one of them was a VJ. Top guy. He told me he'd played football himself at a reasonable level. As we got along well, I invited him and the rest of the crew for a night out with a few of my teammates.

They'd heard a few of my stories about Russian women, so they said yes immediately. I took them to one of my regulars, the Arena Club on Kirpichniy. Loaded with supermodels, and a brilliant VIP area where you could book your own table. The table came with a private toilet – and a curtain. Handy!

Depending on the type of evening, a table cost somewhere between 1,000 and 3,000. Euros, not roubles! But it came with complimentary food and drinks, and they provided you with your own waiter. Top service.

By then, everybody knew me there: the girls behind the bar, the bouncers, the owner even. So there was no need to queue.

It was paradise. What, I've used that word before? But it was, dear reader! The women were triple A category – its dancers and female customers – beyond imagination.

Zenit's two South Koreans agreed on that. I had decided to take them with me, as they were too shy to ask themselves. So, up until I took care of them, the two guys had stayed at home, every single night. Nobody cared about them. Nobody but me.

Before this night, I had taken them on a few introductory trips, first of all to Maximus. I think it was the first time in their lives that they'd come face to face with a stripper. I still remember them going crazy as those naked girls were sitting on their laps. They started some kind of a tap dance, which almost brought tears to my eyes.

Since then, they would be in the club within half an hour of my phone call. They became insatiable. One night, I even gave them two chicks as a takeaway – to enjoy at home. A blonde one and a dark one. 'Thank you, thank you, thank you!' they said.

So I gave them the key to my apartment – like I did with so many other (married) teammates. I didn't have any problems with that – after all, Graciela was never around – but it did mean that I constantly had Zenit players in my house. One of our goalkeepers slept at my place at least three times a week! Although he wasn't sleeping . . .

So, the Koreans had their little private party in my not so humble abode. Later on, I heard they enjoyed their treats so much, that they had swapped after round one. Well, bless them.

Rewind to that night at the Arena, with the MTV crew. I could see my friend getting very nervous. All those wild and willing women I had been talking about . . . he couldn't see any.

He couldn't see them? Well, he noticed their beauty, but he didn't think they were flirting, at least not with him. I told him he was blind. 'Look at those blonde babes over there! Can't you see they're constantly staring at us?'

182

I stood up, walked towards them, and gave one of them a VIP lounge bracelet. Now she belonged to us. 'And you're gonna sit next to *him*!' I said, pointing towards my flabbergasted friend.

That's Russian etiquette for you. They're easy to deal with. Easier than in Scotland or the Netherlands. Yup, they're gold-diggers, but I don't blame them for that. It's their way to get out of their relative poverty. So if you're a rich *and* good-looking guy, you can do anything.

By now, the guy had got it. He waved over at me. 'Can you get the other one for me too?'

'No problem, mate.' I went fishing for the other beauty, who now joined him as well. And off he went. Not with one, but with two top prizes.

For me, Russia was the Land of Sex. Okay, I was still married to Graciela, but she was never there. She hated the place. Most of the time she was in Alkmaar or in our house in Valencia, which we'd bought so that she could be closer to her Spanish family. It was a beautiful place with a pool, not far from the sea, but I was hardly there. Too many obligations in Russia!

I have to confess that I was glad that Graciela wasn't with me in Saint Petersburg. It gave me a lot of freedom. Especially after I changed the Corinthia Nevsky Palace Hotel for my own apartment. At 5,000 euros a month it didn't come cheap, but it was better than living in a hotel. I could bring home one female after the other without getting dirty looks from the hotel staff. I didn't like that any more. It was one of the reasons I moved out.

The new flat was close to the Arena, Nevsky Prospekt, the city's main shopping street, and the Hermitage. Although the museum wasn't the reason I picked it, let's be honest. I know millions of tourists visit the place, to enjoy art created by the likes of Vincent van Gogh, Rembrandt, Picasso, Leonardo da Vinci and Michelangelo, but it wasn't my thing. I was inside the place once, and walked out within minutes. Boring as hell. I have other interests, so to speak.

Eating sushi in the trendy Zima Leto Bar, for instance. And drinking . . . Fanta. Yes, the anti-alcohol vaccination was still in my system, so I couldn't have booze without getting sick as a dog. I didn't mind, didn't miss it at all. Sometimes people asked me if I missed drinking a glass of beer, but I never found it weird when somebody ordered a coffee, so why feel sorry for me and my Fanta?

In the meantime I had developed another addiction: watching people. Okay, watching female people, to be more precise. I keep repeating myself – and don't blame me for that – but it was one supermodel after the other walking by. I could see why Gucci, Chanel, Dolce & Gabbana and Louis Vuitton all had shops on Nevsky Prospekt. It's where their clientele goes!

Despite my Fanta, I was on a high every single time I sat there.

Russia grey and poor? Sure, in certain parts, but not here. Not in the centre of Saint Petersburg. This was para . . . No, we've been through that already.

So, yes, I've seen both sides of the country. One day we went to a town just outside Moscow, for a Cup match against a Third Division team. It was like a trip back in time. Holes in the road the size of a bath tub. Wooden houses like something out of the Middle Ages. It took us two full hours to drive no more than 50 kilometres. It was one of those moments in which you realise how privileged you are to be born in Western Europe.

The big cities are different. There's still a shell of grey communist suburbs around them, but they have a rich and colourful nucleus. There's a lot of money going around in places like Moscow and Saint Petersburg. Sitting in the sun on Nevsky Prospekt, sipping my Fanta, I would count ten Hummers within a few minutes.

Russians like to flaunt their wealth. In the beginning, I thought it was ridiculous. Pure arrogance. But soon I got used to it. Didn't even blink my eyes if I saw two armed guys in a restaurant. My initial thought was: there must be a very, very rich Russian in here – one with a lot of money and a lot of enemies. Those bodyguards, each one built like a wardrobe, didn't even bother hiding their weapons. The guns were just lying on the table in front of them.

And it was not just a matter of showing off. They used the bloody things too! Thank God I've never seen it myself, but I've heard the stories about shootings in restaurants. Hence my advice to everybody: please don't bother those filthy rich bastards. If you hit one of them, it's your fault if you're shot down by these gorillas. It's their job.

I must say, I quickly adapted to the Russian lifestyle. Soon I didn't feel embarrassed any more. Throwing money around in a club? No problem. I had plenty of it. Especially after beating a club from the capital. A 10,000-euro bonus wasn't unusual.

I used to spend it in one night.

Much later, I thought to myself, what an enormous waste! But it was the lifestyle there. We would order the most expensive champagne and, I swear, guys would take one swig of the bottle and . . . buy a new one! This wasn't about drinking, it was about showing everybody how much money you had. Madness.

I couldn't drink at the time. But I didn't care, with all those delicious damsels around to distract me. They were a bonus too. What made me most happy were the results on the pitch. The fact that I had signed with a damn good football club. I mean, we wiped them off the grass. All of them! We were the best of Saint Petersburg, the best of Moscow, the best of Russia! And we played at twice the speed I was used to with Rangers. No exaggerating!

It wasn't kick, rush and forget the midfield either, like in Scotland. There was thought behind everything. Only mentality-wise could we improve, but that was a detail. When it came to the noble art of football, we could beat Ajax and PSV 'with two fingers up our nose', as we say back home.

Actually, the Russian teams didn't stand a chance either. That's how we won the title in 2007, 23 years after Zenit's last championship, in the Soviet Union. We won ours in the last game of the season, on 11 November, in an away game at Saturn Moscow. A horrid game, but that didn't affect the celebrations afterwards. Or during the game, for that matter, as we went apeshit after Radek Sirl's opening goal in the fifteenth minute. And what our goalie Vyacheslav Malafeev did that day was pure magic.

Right after the final whistle, I did a Nobby Stiles in front of the dug-out. Yes, I danced! After my titles in Sittard, Alkmaar and

Glasgow, I was now champion of Russia as well! More to the point, I had won titles at every single one of my clubs! How unique is *that*?

Dick's achievement was a great one: now he was one of just eleven managers with championships in three different countries. Among them, big names like Giovanni Trapattoni, Tomislav Ivic, Ernst Happel, Christoph Daum, Vujadin Boskov and Eric Gerets.

The title parties in town were out of this world. I'm sorry to say, but they were bigger and better than those in Glasgow. We were driven through the city centre in an enormous double-decker, accompanied by Ukrainian boxing legend Vladimir Klitschko, and it was like Moses and the parting of the Red Sea – the sea being the people who swarmed on to the streets in order to catch a glimpse of their heroes. They even managed to turn our little ride into an American ticker-tape parade, with pieces of blue and white paper floating down on us.

It was as if all seven million inhabitants of Saint Petersburg had turned up to celebrate. Unforgettable!

It had been the first time a club from outside Moscow had won the title in the Russian Premjer-Liga. You could tell from the faces of the people how important that was. They had finally beaten Moscow! I bet a lot of them framed the final table, as there was Saint Petersburg at the number one spot and beneath us, in this order, Spartak Moscow, CSKA Moscow, FC Moscow, Saturn Moscow, Dynamo Moscow and Lokomotiv Moscow!

I was proud to be part of the team that achieved that. Okay, due to my Achilles tendon injury I had only played fourteen games that season, but still. You lose together, and you win together.

Same feeling I had after that memorable night in Manchester, in 2008, when we won the UEFA Cup against, of all clubs, Glasgow Rangers. I didn't play one single minute in that final and in the build-up I'd only managed to be active in three games, but still I felt part of the winning team. The medal UEFA chairman Michel Platini gave me that evening, in Manchester City's stadium, was *mine*.

A consolation prize, the UEFA Cup? Get lost! Maybe if you're used to winning the Champions League ten years in a row. But for normal people it's a fantastic trophy.

Right after defeating Villarreal, in the third round, I felt we were going to win the cup. We were like a well-oiled machine. A machine that, later on in the tournament, eliminated Olympique Marseille, Bayer Leverkusen and, in the semi-final, Bayern Munich.

Now, that's what they call being on form!

It hadn't been that easy in the qualification round though. We had a 1–1 against AZ, then being trained by the great Louis van Gaal, and we lost 1–0 to Everton. We really thought it would end there, but AZ were eaten by the Toffeemen too (2–3), so we stayed one point ahead of the cloggies. Together with Everton and 1. FC Nürnberg we reached the next stage of the competition.

The semi-final against Bayern was the highlight, without a doubt. Beating them 4–0, thanks to goals by Pavel Pogrebnyak (two), Konstantin Zyryanov and Viktor Fayzulin, does say something in international football. And after the 1–1 in Bavaria it was: auf Wiedersehen, Fritz!

The home game against Bayern was probably our best one ever. Too bad I was suspended. And, no, it wasn't a second-rate team who faced us, despite the fact that they'd won the German title a few days earlier. Allow me to mention a few names: Franck Ribéry, Bastian Schweinsteiger, Philipp Lahm, Oliver Kahn, Luca Toni, Zé Roberto, Miroslav Klose and Mark van Bommel. Not your average pub team, is it?

And it was wonderful to bump into my old buddy Mark van Bommel. Sixteen years earlier we'd both played in the Fortuna youth team. Who on earth would have expected that all those years later the two of us would play each other in the semi-final of the UEFA Cup? We'd talked about it at the time, playing on the highest international level, but thinking that our dreams would come true and the reality are two different things.

Anyway, I had been a bit worried, the night of the final in Manchester. We had a wonder team, for sure, but as soon as the Russians had to play somewhere across the border, it was as if all of a sudden they were paralysed. I've rarely seen players as good as Andrey Arshavin and Roman Pavlyuchenko, but away from home they were . . . well, not so good. Look how little they achieved later on, at renowned clubs like Arsenal and Tottenham Hotspur. It was as if they couldn't do without their friends, their family and their daily portion of Russian food. I've seen with my own eyes that they didn't even go out at night when we played abroad. Back home they did every godforsaken thing; abroad they seemed to be scared shitless.

Personally, I shouldn't have been worried about Rangers as an opponent. Okay, they had beaten Fiorentina in the semi-final, but they weren't too impressive. Their road to the final had been paved with negative football. Thanks to their manager Walter Smith they had been the cowards of the competition. All games ended in scores like 0–0, 1–0 or 1–1. Boring, boring, boring . . . For your information, our Pavel Pogrebnyak, with ten goals the top scorer of the tournament, had produced more goals than the whole of Glasgow Rangers!

The only weird thing about the final result was that it ended at 2–0 (with goals by Denisov and Zyryanov). We could have hammered them! Nevertheless, it was a memorable game for Zenit, and for Russia. President Vladimir Putin himself phoned Dick while we were in the dressing room. Normally the president has an assistant who makes his phone calls. Not this time, though. Which shows how important the result was for the country.

I was in tears that night. Although I hadn't played at all, I was very emotional. There and then, in the stadium of Manchester City, minutes after the final whistle of the European Cup Final between Rangers and Zenit, I found out that, after all, it is possible to have such a thing as friendship in the totally anti-social world of professional football! Before the game I'd talked to former teammates like Nacho Novo, Allan McGregor and Kris Boyd. We laughed and wished each other success. And after the game, the mutual respect was still there. I remember hugging Jim Bell, Rangers' good old kitman, who was really happy for me, despite the fact that his own team had lost. And, no, he wasn't bullshitting! I didn't think twice when he asked me for my shirt. How could you say no to a lovely chap like Jim?

So, a great evening among old friends and completely different from the times I had to play against AZ. Not so much in October 2007, as things were settled by then. No, I'm talking about the meetings before, when I was still defending the colours of Glasgow Rangers. December 2004, once again in the UEFA Cup tournament.

We had to go to Alkmaar. In the days prior to the confrontation José Fortes Rodriguez – remember him? – told everyone and his dog that Ricksen wasn't welcome any more. According to him, I was the least respectful person he had ever met in his entire life. In the same interview, with Dutch weekly *Sportweek*, Barry van Galen even called me 'an imbecile' who wanted to fight with everybody. And, yes, out came that crappy old story again about me kicking the shit out of Barry Opdam during a training session. Digging the dirt, saying how Opdam was bleeding and how he had cried.

I laughed about it. At the time, Opdam had been an adult. And adults don't cry after a little clash, do they? Besides, it had been self-defence.

Still, the words of Rodriguez kept jogging through my mind, as if on a treadmill. No respect? Who is showing no respect here? You, Rodriguez! What had I done? I hadn't stolen your money – nor your girlfriend. I had just shown a winner's mentality.

Hmmm, maybe he was still pissed off about the fact that girls in general fancied me more than him . . . That could be it. Frustration, maybe.

Anyway, no wobbly knees that night in Alkmaar. And, indeed, nothing happened. It had been all mouth and no trousers. Just a pity that we lost that night: 1–0, with a goal by Denny Landzaat, who would end up at Wigan Athletic. We were the better team, but we ended up empty-handed. Eventually we found ourselves in fourth position, behind AZ, AJ Auxerre and Grazer AK, which for us meant the end of the tournament.

But years later I had the honour of visiting the Kremlin, as part of the team that had won that cup. After CSKA Moscow in 2005 we were only the second Russian team to lay its hands on that prize. The Russian PM Dmitri Medvedev, himself a huge Zenit fan, wanted to thank us in person. Ukrainian president Viktor Yushchenko, the leader of the Russian Orthodox church and the boss of the Moscow Patriarchate were other VIPs who wanted to pay their respects to us.

I didn't know how special it was to be invited to the Kremlin until I heard that the Catharina Hall, where we were supposed to meet the PM, was normally only used to invite world leaders, like the President of the United States. So, yes, this time I was nervous! I was about to shake the hand of one of the most powerful people on the globe. And where would I do that? In a room where people like Ronald Reagan and Bill Clinton had stood. Not bad for a street kid from Hoensbroek!

My first thought when I saw Medvedev entering the room: what a small guy! Of course the other little fella, Dick Advocaat, was the first one he shook hands with. Much later, after the PM had told us how proud he was, there was a handshake for me too. It was very impressive.

Sometimes people ask me: why didn't you pull back your hand, Fernando? You're such a big prankster. It would've made great TV!

No, not this time. Too much respect.

Too bad I've never met Vladimir Putin, who was born in Saint Petersburg. Dick has. The two became acquaintances. Putin used to call Dick to wish him a happy birthday and even gave him birthday presents; one time, a beautiful and very expensive watch. Quite a contrast to the chocolate ball Zenit gave him, when he turned 59 . . .

Putin is the absolute number one person in Russia. You don't get them more powerful than him. The times we had to stay up in the air above Moscow, because Putin was on the ground and we were not allowed to land until he had gone . . .

Medvedev wasn't the last VIP we would meet. After our visit to the Kremlin, we had an audition at the Mariinsky Palace with the mayor of Saint Petersburg, Valentina Matvienko. Once again it was a memorable moment, not least for Dick, who was made Honorary Citizen of Saint Petersburg, the first foreign one since 1866. The rest of us were given inviolability.

I kid you not.

From that moment on I was inviolable. The chief inspector of Saint Petersburg, the very same one whose number was in Arshavin's mobile phone, told us. Inviolability. I would never have to worry about the police again.

Unheard of in the Netherlands. Nobody would accept that. But this was Russia. And in Russia, anything's possible. And not a single politician would object.

From that moment on I was more or less invincible. I didn't have to pay cops any more; nobody could make me do anything. And you know what? I didn't even feel embarrassed!

SIXTEEN

DOWNHILL

THE CHANGES DICK MADE at Zenit and the structure he laid down were bearing fruit. We were winning more and more silverware. For instance, the European Super Cup, on 29 August 2008, in the Stade Louis II in Monaco. This was unique, as since the mighty Soviet Union had fallen to pieces not a single Russian club had achieved that.

And who did we beat? Manchester United! Yup, the very same Red Devils who'd won the Champions League a few months earlier. The Big United, so to say, with hot shots like Edwin van der Sar, Wayne Rooney, Rio Ferdinand, Patrice Evra, Carlos Tévez, Paul Scholes and Nani. And they were all playing against us, as Alex Ferguson refused to look upon the confrontation as a summer night's friendly. Served him right. Anyone who treats a European cup as a minor prize is a nutcase.

For Fergie there was even more at stake. Given the fact that he had won the trophy already in 1983 and 1991, this would be his third time as manager – and that would make him the first one ever! Hence the extremely strong line-up he put on the pitch that day.

Ferguson's opponent in the other corner, Little General Advocaat, wanted to win the damn thing too. Dick wants to win everything, even a game of Monopoly. More to the point, he knew he would be judged by the amount of prizes he would win with Zenit – prizes and nothing else. The Russian Super Cup, which we'd grabbed before the eyes of Lokomotiv Moscow a few weeks earlier, was one of those goblets.

It wasn't an easy clash, the one with Man Utd. From the very first second the Mancunians were on the attack. But we held our ground, despite big chances from Rooney and Tévez. And after a while the game started to tilt in our favour. Exactly as Dick wanted. From then on, it was a matter of waiting – waiting for the first Zenit goal.

And soon it was there. And a second one too. First was a header by Pavel Pogrebnyak, in the 45th minute of the game, and then an individual masterpiece from Danny, the little Portuguese dribbler we'd bought from Dynamo Moscow only four days ago.

Dick saw that the game and the cup were ours, so he sat back, relaxed, as if he was watching, er, a football match on TV. Eventually United managed to make it 2–1 – with a goal by defender Nemanja Vidic – but it was too late for them. Zenit won the Super Cup.

Zenit was ready to dominate, like Manchester United, AC Milan, Real Madrid and Barcelona had done before. Zenit was at the gates of Europe. Nobody could ignore us any more.

I didn't play that night. That bloody Achilles tendon was still bothering me. There was a 'floating' piece of bone in my ankle, or so the doctors had told me. Anyway, Dick didn't want to take any risks. He only used players that were 100 per cent fit. I couldn't blame him for that, but I was extremely pissed off. It hurt – in more than one way.

But, as the mighty Johan Cruyff once said: every disadvantage has its advantage. Being off the chalk board meant that I didn't have to prepare for the game, so I could leave the Riviera Marriott Hotel La Porte de Monaco and go into town.

I, Fernando Ricksen from Little Chicago, was in Monte Carlo, a diamond's throw away from the most famous nightclub in the world, Jimmy'z, on the Avenue Princesse Grace, where a cheap bottle of wine costs you 600 euros and where only the extremely rich and famous come to party. I'd heard so many stories about the place . . . and now I was here. This was a once in a lifetime experience.

So I went, together with my Belgian buddy Nicolas Lombaerts, who we had bought from AA Gent the previous year. He was injured too. Worse than me even: he was on crutches. He said he didn't feel like dancing anyway. And as 'kruk' in Dutch means both 'crutch' and 'stool', for him it was just a matter of changing one kruk for the other.

I joined him at the bar. And not for an overpriced Fanta this time. I was on the sauce again. The injection I'd had in the summer of 2006 wasn't working any more. I had found out one day in Valencia when I had ordered a virgin sangria and, by mistake, the waiter had supplied me with a real one.

After two gulps of the fruity stuff, it was like a funfair inside my head. Alcohol! I got scared. I thought about the consequences it would have for my body. I was going to be as sick as a dog, for sure, because Manuel from *Fawlty Towers* had made a bloody mistake! *Que?*

So I waited for the inevitable to happen. But it didn't. No red spots, no puking. After ten minutes nothing had happened, and I felt great. The vaccination wasn't working any more! What a wonderful day!

I could hit the booze again – and, boy, had I missed it! Despite all the problems I'd had with the poison, I couldn't wait to have it back in my veins again.

So, back to the bar at Jimmy'z, where the two of us had found a good spot . . . It'll take a big boy to drag me away from here, I said to myself. And we started drinking, Nicolas and me. Non-stop. Until the lights went off. Inside me, that is, not inside Jimmy'z.

A few minutes later – or so I thought – my first thought was for Nicolas. After all, he was on crutches. What if he fell flat on his face? Fernando would be to blame, for sure. So I had to get him out of the place as fast as possible.

Outside, I asked for a taxi. Twice, probably, as by then I was seeing double. The cab arrived faster than expected, I opened the door, threw Nicolas inside, and shouted, 'See ya at breakfast!'

Yes, I stayed. This was Jimmy'z, people! I knew I would regret it later if I left then. So bye bye Nicolas, watch those crutches! And back into Jimmy'z I went. Back to the supermodels and, er, the drinks.

My first mistake of the night. The second came shortly afterwards, as I downed a glass of strong wine as if it was water. Combined with the heat, this was an absolute killer. I blacked out.

You stupid fucker, Ricksen! Get out of this place *now*!

Seconds later, I was on the doorstep of Jimmy'z, enjoying the fresh Mediterranean sea breeze. Enough of this stupid drinking, I wanted to get to my bed in the Marriott – and I wanted to get there fast.

Just one problem. *Where* exactly was the bloody bed? I was too drunk to remember the way back to the hotel. And there were no cabs at that time of night. I could have asked the bouncers or any passer-by where the hotel was, but I was too dumb to think about that.

Now I did something extremely stupid: I started to walk. After all, the hotel was nearby, wasn't it? But did I have to turn left or right? Right, I said to myself.

Wrong.

After an hour of fruitless wandering, I still hadn't found the Marriott. Nor any other hotel. Nor *anything*, for that matter!

I was out in the sticks. All I could see was a petrol station, and it was closed. I decided to sit there and wait. The people from the petrol station would open the place within an hour, for sure. And they could help me. The stupidest thing to do would be to walk any further, in this mountainous environment. That would only make my situation a lot worse. As if that was possible!

It wouldn't be too good for my ankle either. I'd already fallen a few times – and my clothes were ripped. What a mess!

Sitting near the petrol station, I fought to stay awake – a fight that I lost. I fell asleep on the tarmac, my last thought being: let's hope Nicolas got home safely.

So there I was, fast asleep, near an abandoned petrol station, in ripped clothes and with red wine stains all over my white shirt. I've had better moments, I can assure you.

Eventually two cops woke me up and asked me what I was doing there. Hmmm, good question. One I couldn't answer. *Dick!* What would he say if the coppers took me to the police station, a few hours before the most important game in Zenit's club history? Dick would freak out. He didn't know I was out and he didn't know I was drinking again.

I don't know how or in which language exactly, but I managed to convince the policemen of the fact that I wasn't a tramp, rather I was a lost football player who needed to get to his bed in the Marriott Hotel.

And that is exactly where they took me, in their police car. It was the highlight of the evening. And I don't think Dick ever found out.

Still, I was a bit worried when I entered the hotel that morning in my Worzel Gummidge outfit, as I bumped into the four UEFA officials who had been in Monaco to guide us. I walked as straight as possible to the elevator, hoping they wouldn't say anything to my manager.

It was eight in the morning. Breakfast was served at nine . . . Not even a cold shower could freshen me up. I was sick as a parrot and pissed as a dog – or the other way around – and my eyes were as red as the tomatoes in the breakfast buffet. Through half-shut lids, I could see Dick's angry face. But I decided to ignore it.

To convince everybody I was feeling fine, I took an extra cheese roll and a nice glass of milk, and kept smiling. Say cheese!

After breakfast I immediately went back to my room. I crashed out and slept for the rest of the day, until I had to go to the stadium and watch the game.

Later that night, things went downhill again – at, er, Jimmy'z . . .

This time we were there with the entire squad. Some rich Russians had hired the club, and once again money was no object. They'd even flown in some of Russia's most famous DJs. But I couldn't keep my head up. I was still knackered from the previous night. So I left the place at two. By taxi, this time.

A few days later, in Saint Petersburg, I got drunk again. And the day after. And the day after . . . you guessed it. But it was worse than in Scotland. I wasn't drinking because I liked it. I was drinking because I needed it. I had become a full-blown alcoholic.

One of the reasons for hitting the bottle was the fact that I was hardly playing. At times I wasn't even included in the squad. For the first time in my entire career I was left out of the team structure. I had to channel the anger that came with it – and I did it with alcohol.

At that point, my life was in turmoil. Everything collided: my injury, the fact that I wasn't part of the team any more, my imminent divorce from Graciela . . . I simply couldn't handle it. Sometimes I stayed at home, deliberately, so that I wouldn't drink anything. But it didn't work. I couldn't relax at all. On the contrary, within minutes I was totally stressed out. That's because I realised what a mess I'd made of my life – and that of others. Those thoughts led to a headache, which I had to kill with booze.

Alcohol turned out to be my only medicine. The pain in my head would disappear and I would have fun again. But by this stage I wasn't sitting on my own sofa, I was in the Arena Club. Just to inform you.

In the Arena there were still people around me who gave me the impression that they admired me. As if I were king. I was the centre of attention – always. And it was a fantastic feeling. Every night people wanted to enter the Arena with me. At first I said no, as I still had to play the odd game of football. But after a while, that barrier had gone. So I said yes. Always.

Who cared that Zenit had a match coming up? I certainly didn't! I always joined friends on a trip downtown. And if nobody asked me I would invite them! They always said yes, as I was constantly waving my credit card around. And thanks to me they visited places they would never see otherwise, with their normal wage packets. I knew every bouncer in Saint Petersburg, so nobody ever had to queue up.

On nights like that, I spent thousands of pounds. And this went on for weeks, if not months. Now, looking back, I think how incredibly stupid it was. But back then, I simply didn't recognise the value of money. Thanks to my salary, I was living in a bubble.

Money was also the root of my downfall. I sometimes think that if I hadn't had all that cash, things might have been better. But who knows?

Due to the fact that I now had one *ouch* after the other, I very rarely played a game. In 2008 I made eight appearances, most of them as a substitute. In 2009, zero. Zilch. And I still made truckloads of money.

It made me depressed. So I took the next step into hell. In order to feel better I now turned to drugs. Booze on its own didn't do the trick any more.

Drugs were they only way I could get sober again. Well, sort of . . .

I wasn't new to dope. Back in my younger days, I'd seen a lot of kids doing it in the street. In the bars and clubs of Alkmaar, the stuff was available too. I did pop the occasional pill in those days, but never during the season. Only when I didn't have to play. I was too scared to get caught.

Back in Heerlerheide it was easy getting a few pills. Everybody knew where to get them and it was a pretty druggy neighbourhood. In Saint Petersburg I didn't have to search for them either. There was just one big difference from my drugs consumption in the past: this time I was swallowing pills during the season as well.

Now, talk about taking risks . . . I took a *huge* shot in the dark here. But I didn't care. It was now my way of surviving. And it wasn't just pills. Because of the shit I was in, I started shoving Charlie up my nose too. Yup, cocaine. Complimentary stuff from some Russian gangsters I'd befriended.

I was going more and more off the rails. Not that I snorted the stuff every day. Sometimes my nose was coke-free for weeks! I only used it when I needed it, although I admit that during my last months in Russia I needed it a *lot*. But I still didn't see myself as an addict.

I did like the stuff though. And so did my hangers-on. People say the guys around me were taking advantage of me. I saw it the other way around: I was taking advantage of them. I was buying fun and attention off them.

Suicide wasn't an option. Are you kidding me? My life was in pieces, but thanks to the coke and the booze and the cash and the girls I still had a hell of a time. I was having heaps of fun. And when I felt sad, say after another useless training session, I just went to bed. When I was asleep everything was fine. After I woke up, late afternoon, reality would kick in. But then I would take a drink – and soon I'd feel like a million dollars again.

Not an ideal lifestyle for a professional footballer, I can hear you say . . .

In the meantime I had befriended Maja, Macha, Anna and Viktoria, four gorgeous strippers from club Maximus. I even gave them the key to my apartment, which, as you may remember, happened to be situated right around the corner from the strip joint. It gave them the opportunity to drop in, even when I wasn't at home. It was for practical reasons: they lived in the outskirts which are hardly reachable in the middle of the night. In order to let ships through on the river Neva, all bridges are up by then. If you really have to get back to your place, you have to take the ring road. Additional driving time: *three hours*. So, it was better for the girls to stay at my place and wait for the bridges to come down.

Needless to say they came quite often. Especially in the morning, after they'd finished work. In the end, they moved in. By then I didn't even see them as pole dancers. They were, well, my friends. Not girlfriends though, as I was still married to Graciela. I didn't have a relationship with any of the dancers – or any other Russian girl, for that matter.

Still, I loved to have them around. Top girls they were – and nutters too. They were crazy! What sane girl wants to be a pole dancer? That was probably why we all got along so well. I was a nutcase too!

In between lodging, they did a bit of shopping for me, cleaned the apartment and prepared food. They accompanied me when I had to buy a new phone card, or do something at the bank. They were my perfect personal assistants.

Obviously they disappeared when Graciela dropped by.

Did I ever have sex with those goddesses? Of course! Picture this: the strip club closes, the dancers come home full of adrenaline, they see me sleeping, jump into bed with me and . . . Would you say no in that situation? Would you send them away? I bet you wouldn't!

Still, they weren't around just for sex. I had other girls for that. Girls I picked up at the clubs in Saint Petersburg. No, they weren't hookers. I don't do hookers. Apart from that one time in South Africa, I've never paid for sex. I could get the best women for free. A thousand euros for an hour, those Russian prostitutes cost. I preferred to spend that on champagne, to tell you the truth. Besides, sex with a whore isn't fun. A working girl only keeps an eye on her watch. I detest that. I like the whole process of chatting up, having a laugh et cetera.

That's why things worked out so well with the Maximus girls. We did a lot of things together, apart from having sex. On their nights off, I sometimes took them out to a restaurant. Oh, I loved the dirty looks some of the players' wives gave us when they saw us entering Loge.

I preferred to take my girls there, because I knew a few of my colleagues' partners would be there too. The faces they pulled when they saw me entering the place with not one, not two, not three, but *four* drop-dead gorgeous women . . .

The players who were there with their partners showed signs of disapproval too. In reality, I think they envied me.

I loved it. Other people loved it too. Like a Dutch friend who came to visit me one day. As he arrived quite late, I took him straight from Pulkovo Airport to the Arena Club. I hadn't told him about my lodgers yet. Some things are best kept secret, at least for a while.

As Russian vodka is stronger than the stuff we have back home, the liquid KO'd him quite fast, so I had to drag him home and pour him into bed.

The next morning I got up early because I had to go to training. As a hardened boozer, I didn't feel like a wreck at all. I could handle the alcohol better than Arshavin, who, as you may remember, fell over the ball on my very first training session in Russia. I wasn't like that. Fighting Spirit in the bar, Fighting Spirit on the pitch.

After the training session I switched on my mobile and saw that

I had ten missed calls! All made by my legless friend back home. Something was wrong! I called him immediately.

He sounded upset. 'Fernando, please . . .'

'Yes?'

'Please, tell me . . . which brothel am I in?'

'Brothel? What do you mean?'

'Which brothel did you dump me in, Fernando? It's full of chicks wearing nothing but G-strings. What did you do? Get me out of here!'

'Oh . . . That's my home, actually. And those girls are my friends Maja, Macha, Anna and Viktoria. Don't panic, they won't do you any harm!'

As I entered my house, a bit later, I saw him sitting on my sofa. To his left were Macha and Anna, and to his right were Maja and Viktoria. He looked as if he ruled the place. The new Tsar of Saint Petersburg.

Each girl knew the city like the back of her hand and this meant that, thanks to them, I ended up in places the average foreigner never would. So on a night in August . . .

Yes, this is the beginning of yet another tale.

Normally I never left the centre of Saint Petersburg. Way too dangerous! What if I went home with a girl, only to be confronted by an armed husband? Try to escape? Try to survive, more like!

I didn't want to take that risk. So, unlike in Glasgow, I always took my girl back to my own den. I also told my mates where I would be that night. Safety first. For that reason I had my personal cab driver too. He would wait all night until I staggered out of a club.

But, for once, on a beautiful summer night, I changed my pattern and decided to have a look outside the centre. So when my flatmates asked me, giggling, if I wanted to go 'somewhere nice', I said yes. I trusted the girls like my own wallet. No, more than that!

Off we went, in one of their cars, towards the Gulf of Finland. And it was then that I started to have doubts. It was getting darker and darker, the roads were getting worse and worse, and I didn't like the idea any more. I felt, sort of, scared. I didn't know where I was, didn't know what to expect.

I imagined myself being tied up, the culmination of a project the girls had been working on for months. Think about that scene in *Reservoir Dogs* . . .

Why oh why had I agreed to this? Why had I put myself into this vulnerable position? You dickhead! And why hadn't I told anybody that we were heading out of the city? What if they were going to shoot me? Would they ever find my body in this remote part of the country?

I couldn't get these nasty thoughts out of my mind. Started sweating. Outside, it was pitch black. Nobody would be able to trace me here. I thought about the one million ransom they would ask for me. This had happened to foreigners before. How the fuck was I going to get out of this car?

I took a close look at the girls' faces. No signs of stress. They were still in a really good mood, as they always were. It was time to pop the question.

'Where are we going to?'

They didn't answer. Instead, I saw index fingers being pressed firmly against lovely lips. 'No.' And, 'Don't worry, it's gonna be all right.' And, 'You'll be amazed.'

When we finally stopped we'd almost reached the Finnish border. In front of us was a huge mansion bathed in floodlights. Inside, the music was so loud that we could hear it from outside.

This was the girls' surprise. I had been taken to one of Russia's most exclusive nightclubs as a VIP. It was their way of saying thank you for all those months of love and care.

Now, wasn't that sweet of them? Yes, it was. Still, I swore to myself that I would never put myself into a situation like that again.

Adventures like that made my life a rollercoaster. Things were never predictable with me. I loved the excitement, the tension and, in hindsight, the danger.

Completely at odds with my professional life. Since the summer of 2008, when the boys won the European Super Cup, I'd been training for nothing. My main rivals on the right wing, Anyukov and Denisov, were fitter than me. I had great difficulties with the situation, as any footballer would. Since 26 October 2008 in Siberia

– Tom Tomsk away, always difficult – I hadn't played a single match.

Still, I had a contract so I had to show up at the training sessions. And I did – I was still a professional, you know. And I did what Dick told me to do, whether I agreed with it or not. It wasn't like what happened at Fortuna once, many years ago, when Richard Sneekes refused to go on the pitch in injury time. Manager Chris Dekker wanted to use him as a last-minute substitute, but Sneekes told him to fuck off and said that the 90 minutes had gone already.

I was astounded. How could a player say a thing like that to his manager? I would never have done that, no matter how humiliating a manager's decision was.

Sometimes Dick totally forgot about me when I was doing my warm-up during the game. But it wasn't out of disrespect; it was because he was so focused on the match itself. I could have waved like a windmill and he still wouldn't have noticed me.

This didn't happen when we played Amkar Perm, somewhere in the Urals. After twenty minutes of stretching and running, I was told to go on. It was ridiculous, as the clock in the stadium had stopped already. There were only a few seconds left. So, it would basically take the rhythm out of the game. I thought it was an insult to an experienced footballer of 32 years of age. C'mon, is this what you took me with you for? Two five-hour flights and a night in a dodgy hotel for this? Why don't you use a youngster instead?

Cor Pot left, immediately after winning the UEFA Cup. He was made head coach of the Dutch national youth team and, according to him, it was time to be his own boss again. It was an emotional moment for me, as Cor and I had become close friends. But it was an offer he couldn't refuse, he told me. Still, it was sad. Bye, Cor, lover of beautiful buildings and even more beautiful women! Old scamp, I still remember you showing me your phone with a pic of your latest catch – usually a blonde.

I wasn't surprised that he was so popular among the female population of Saint Petersburg. Well groomed men are real babe magnets over there. Just ask, er, me!

SEVENTEEN

COLLISION COURSE

AT SOME STAGE, DICK lost it. His grip, that is. He was still the boss, but not that much of a general any more. He couldn't get the team to play the way he wanted any longer. It was as if we were over the hill. Even Denisov, the future captain of the Russian team, wasn't as good as in our super season.

This was partly due to the fact that our big star Arshavin had left. After nine years with Zenit he finally chose Arsenal. The Gunners paid more than 20 million euros for him. At an earlier stage, Barcelona found that sum too high. I was happy for my teammate, but he would have done better in Spain, in my opinion.

So there we were, without Andrey. Sure, there were still enough other good players, but none of them was as brilliant as him. He was a weirdo, but a genius, a magician. I wasn't surprised when, a few weeks after his departure, he scored four times against Liverpool. At Anfield!

Anyway, this left us without a real leader on the pitch. As a team we were a lot less without him. Just look at the table: halfway through 2009 we were seventh, miles behind later champions Rubin Kazan. A disgrace for a club like Zenit.

Not that I needed to mention this to Dick. He knew it. Time was running out for him. He did his best, together with Cor Pot's successor Bert van Lingen, but the magic had disappeared. After a 0–2 defeat against Tom Tomsk, the Little General was given his marching orders. The date: 10 August 2009. Our next boss would be Anatoliy Davydov, up until then coach of Zenit's reserves.

Our bad results weren't the only reason for Dick's dismissal though. The hot shots at Zenit were not amused by the fact that he had made a deal with the Belgian FA, without telling them. As from January, Dick would be – hold on, here comes a word play! – the Red Devils' Advocaat.

Oh, and Dick had become a victim of defamation, thanks to that scumbag Radimov. I've no idea what he told the board behind Dick's back, but it wasn't a eulogy! Radimov had a few collaborators, as he wasn't man enough to do things on his own, but they succeeded, those traitors, and Dick had to leave the club.

I was out of my mind with rage when I heard it. This was the final nail in the coffin. I got very emotional when I heard about it. At that point, I'd had it with Zenit. Completely. Okay, I could have thought, maybe a new manager will give me a chance, as with Dick at the helm I hadn't been playing anyway. After all, hadn't I had my best period with Rangers after Dick's departure? On top of that, I still had a contract and the prospect of earning 1.2 million euros clear, for doing a bit of stretching on the training ground and spending 90 minutes on the bench every weekend. Easy money, eh?

Yes, easy money, but blood money at the same time. I couldn't stand the idea of sharing a dressing room with a bunch of crooks who had stabbed Dick in the back. He was, and always will be, a kind, warm personality who deserved better than that.

Much better! Dick deserved a statue! Or a job as technical director. But for that position Zenit had contracted former Feyenoord and Barcelona player Igor Korneev. Dick couldn't stand the guy and I understood why.

At the end of July Korneev had bought an Italian, Alessandro Rosina. The guy was a midfielder from Torino. A good player, but Dick hadn't asked for him. Nor had Belarus-born Sergei Kornilenko been on his wish list. Dick wanted Goran Pandev from Macedonia. And Peruvian Paolo Guerrero. But he didn't get them, and it was the start of a battle the Little General couldn't win.

I won't deny it: things were going downhill at Zenit. A fifth spot in 2008 and a seventh by the time Dick was kicked out in 2009. But the entire foundation the club had been rebuilt on was laid down by one man: Dick Advocaat. And all the titles – the UEFA Cup, the European Super Cup and the Russian Super Cup – had been the work of that very same little chap, one who had been proclaimed Russian Coach of the Year. And now they had kicked him out. Bloody cowards.

At least he was given a decent send-off. After a game, he was driven round the stadium in an open Bentley. Dick, being the emotional man he is, had to wipe the tears from his eyes.

Despite that memorable tribute, I wanted to force a decision – a fracture, more to the point. It wouldn't be too difficult, as everyone knew I was back on the booze. Bert van Lingen and Dutch physiotherapist Rob Ouderland tried to help me, but I didn't accept their support. I told them I didn't have any problems, and even if I did, I would be man enough to deal with them. I was reacting as I had in my worst days in Scotland. And further downhill I went . . .

In the eyes of Zenit, I was a member of Team Dick – a friend of the enemy. So after the departure of Dick (and Bert and Rob), I knew I was close to being kicked out as well. I didn't have to wait long. On 23 August, just two weeks after Dick got sacked, I was forced to leave too.

It was actually a minor incident that triggered it. As I lived next door to the hotel where Zenit always stayed in the hours before a match, I regularly went home in between. I ate at the hotel, I slept at the hotel, but come time off, I walked to my house. I had always done that. I didn't see the problem. We were free to do whatever we wanted, so why not stay at my own place for a while? And I always kept an eye on the clock, always. I respected the club rules.

Dick never made an issue out of it. So surely the new manager wouldn't mind. Or would he?

The next morning I walked straight from my hotel room to the place where breakfast was served. I had a healthy appetite, so I was looking forward to my cheese rolls and stuff. It's just that I never made it to the buffet.

At the bottom of the stairs stood new manager Davydov. Suddenly he started yelling at me. I had no idea why. The previous night I'd been in my room before eleven and I hadn't even been drinking! (I never drank before a match, only before training sessions in the later stages of my alcoholism.)

I knew I had little chance of playing against Lokomotiv Moscow but I had behaved myself. I'd been a good boy, a professional. A few days earlier I'd been part of the squad that travelled to Madeira for a Europa League play-off game against Nacional. I didn't kick a single ball, but I was still there as part of the team. So maybe there was a chance of a performance against Lok Moscow.

Well, until I reached the bottom of the stairs . . . There, I was confronted with an extremely angry Davydov asking me why I hadn't been 'there' the previous night and 'where' I had been. I thought he was taking the Mickey out of me. He knew I had been home. But he went on and on about it, so he must have been deadly serious.

That was it. I snapped. 'Fuck you!' Not very nice, I know, but the words just came out of my mouth. I couldn't keep them in.

'I beg your pardon?'

'Didn't you hear me? Fuck you! Get stuffed! Oh, and rip my contract to pieces at the same time. I'm finished with you lot! Do you understand? *Finished!*'

I didn't care any more, as you may have noticed.

Davydov didn't even look insulted. He just nodded. I think he liked my proposition.

I was free. I didn't even have to show up for the match a few hours later.

So those sixty seconds as a substitute against Amkar Perm, in November 2008, were my last ones for Zenit Saint Petersburg. It was sad that it had to end there, on a crappy ground west of the Urals. I don't even think it was televised. What a way to end a beautiful chapter of my life. Painful.

Later on, I heard that Davydov had only done this to show the rest of the players who was the boss. To assert his authority. Not very honest of him, but, hey, ever heard of karma? By the end of December Davydov had already been replaced! By one Luciano Spalletti, that hairless Herbert from AS Roma. Now *that* was a short and, in all honesty, not so successful career. Or was it, Davydov? They ended third that year, after champions Rubin Kazan. Thinking about it, it was a top result.

My explosion at the bottom of the stairs came as a relief. I didn't regret it at all. Not even the next morning, when I realised my incredibly lucrative contract was in tatters. I was glad I felt that way, because what would have happened if I'd felt sorry about myself? Then, dear reader, I would have had a problem – a big, big problem. Can you imagine me crawling back? Offering my apologies to Davydov? No way! They would have taken the piss out of me big time.

But I didn't want to belong to Zenit any more. It felt wonderful not to belong to *anybody* any more!

In the meantime I had started a relationship with a young Russian girl, Veronika. I knew her from the Arena Club. Now don't get me wrong, she managed the VIP reservations at the venue! At first, I didn't want to develop any feelings for her, as I was still tied to Graciela. But when it became clear that our marriage was over and my sexy lodgers had moved out, I took the risk of dating her. And guess what happened? Too easy. I fell in love with her.

The main difference between Veronika and all the other girls was that she wasn't after my money (money that was getting relatively scarce too, because I was about to become unemployed). Veronika taught me how not to waste cash. Well, even if I had wanted to continue burning banknotes the way I was used to, I couldn't. Because Graciela was plundering our joint bank account to the tune of hundreds of thousands of euros.

So I had to become modest. And I had decided that I didn't want to get back into the dirty world of professional football any more. After twenty years I had had enough. No more fakery, no more lies. No more matches, hotel rooms, training grounds, team gatherings.

It was time to do something completely different – although I didn't have a clue what.

First a nice holiday, I said to myself. Relaxing near my own pool in Valencia. Emptying my head, as they say. That was more important than my future. So that's what I told Veronika. I was scared that it would freak her out, but I was wrong. Rich footballer or not-so-rich job seeker, she didn't give a toss. She chose me for who I was as a human being. That was a first time for me.

As I didn't want to stay in Russia one minute longer than necessary, I terminated my apartment lease and took off. Just like that. Didn't say goodbye to anybody. I took Veronika with me and we spent three weeks at my home in Spain. I unwound completely. I've hardly ever been so happy as I was then. It was much, much better than my usual holidays in the Caribbean. As a footballer, the next season is always in the back of your mind. So, even on vacation, you do a bit of exercising. Now I didn't have to do anything at all. What a luxury!

The happy feeling lasted exactly 21 days. To be exact, until I arrived at Schiphol Airport. There, the police were waiting with a letter. A letter from Graciela. I read it and freaked out. After our divorce, it said, my ex-wife was demanding 60,000 euros from me. Per month! Alimony!

'She's lost it!' I screamed. 'We don't even have a child together!'

No way was I going to do this. No way! She was not going to break my back! It was time to show her some of that good old Fighting Spirit!

It would be the start of a long and hostile battle.

Between Veronika and me, things went from strength to strength. I even asked her to stay with me. I knew it would be better for me, as she acted like a kind of mentor. Thanks to her I didn't do drugs any more. Thanks to her I stopped my excessive drinking. Thanks to her I realised that there was more to life than me, myself and I.

She had tamed me! Or so it seemed.

And there was plenty of room in the Netherlands for my Russian girlfriend. I still had a house in Alkmaar, and one in the outskirts of

Amsterdam, in an area called Osdorp, which we'd bought because it was convenient for the airport.

The place in Osdorp became our love shack. (Graciela was living in the house in Alkmaar, where she'd changed all the locks.) I didn't mind. Amsterdam was fine for me. I could be completely anonymous there. No amateur psychologists bothering me with their well-intended advice. Hey, if I want to play football again, I'll raise the topic myself, okay?

But I didn't. I watched it on TV, but that was it. I didn't miss playing it at all. Not even when I saw guys kicking a ball who were a lot less talented than me. Yes, I was talented – very talented! And you don't forget how to play football, even though you don't train on a regular basis.

I was still in good shape. Just as in my football days I completely rejected junk food like crisps, chips and burgers. No way was I going to flush twenty years of professional training down the toilet. Now that would have been a waste!

I kept in shape by walking and running. All in all I gained four kilos, which was peanuts. If I ever decided to make a comeback, I said to myself, those four kilos would disappear within hours! But, no, I wasn't going to make a comeback. It was a bit strange when the season started though. For the first time in two decades I wasn't sitting in a dressing room. But I got over it very quickly. I had other things on my mind.

I was busy travelling. Showing Veronika the world. We went to Monte Carlo and Italy. We even jumped on the high-speed Thalys to Paris! We had the time of our lives.

The gap between football and me became wider and wider. I didn't even check the results any more, didn't know where Rangers and Zenit were in their respective tables. I just wasn't interested.

It was also because I had a new distraction. A pub of my own. No, not to drink dry, to earn money with! I was going into business! At first – er, you can imagine why – I had my doubts. A friend of mine asked me whether I'd be interested in taking over Se7en, a lounge bar in the heart of Alkmaar. Now, asking an ex-alcoholic to take over a watering hole is like asking for trouble, isn't it? I could hear the jokes already: I would become my own best customer. But I wanted to prove my critics wrong. I saw it as an enormous challenge. I still loved to drink the occasional glass of wine at dinner, but I wouldn't fall into that booze-soaked hell again. Veronika wouldn't let that happen.

So I did it! Without any experience? Well, you can't say I haven't seen a bar from the inside, can you? I'd also demolished a thing or two in the past, as you know from this book, but for Se7en I decided to leave the breaking of the walls to some professionals. I was more the captain of the team, telling them where the counter should be, what colour the walls should be, those kind of things. And, not least, which spirits we were going to serve. That's where my past came in handy . . .

I loved Se7en. I loved it so much that after the opening in 2010 I sometimes acted as a bartender: chatting with the customers, tapping a beer, putting on some music. It was hard work, but it gave me something to do. And it kept me off the hard liquor, just as I wanted.

I felt great.

Okay, it wasn't comparable to the stress before a Champions League match, but I did feel a certain tension. This was my place and I didn't want to ruin my name again, like I'd done so often in the past. I had to stay focused.

But there was no need to worry; the place was a success. Even AZ players, like goalkeeper Esteban, dropped by for a drink. Hats off to them, as I hadn't left the club in particularly good spirits ten years earlier.

Nevertheless, when I wasn't working there myself, the place was almost empty. At least that's what my employees told me. Maybe, I said to myself, people prefer to have a drink at the neighbours', as soon as they see Fernando isn't in. After all, I was a bit of an attraction. A former international football player serving drinks, they kinda liked that. I used to give autographs and pose for photos. Oh, and there was a worldwide financial crisis, let's not forget that element!

So I didn't think much of it. I concentrated on other things, like finding the right DJ for a theme night. Decorating the place with skulls for Halloween. I even had one that made a sound as soon as you walked past it. Hilarious. And I painted the place orange when the national team was playing. My heart still had that colour. Besides, the squad still included a lot of guys I'd played with, like Giovanni van Bronckhorst, Mark van Bommel, Wesley Sneijder, Arjen Robben, Rafael van der Vaart – all former teammates of mine! Guys who even made it to the World Cup final in South Africa! Supervised by Bert van Marwijk, a coach with a Fortuna heart and, not unimportant, father-in-law of my chum Van Bommel! Not a bunch of people you're gonna let down.

And what a final it was. We could have beaten the mighty Spain we were so close. The moment Robben was on his way to the Spanish goalkeeper – a matter of centimetres. But we lost, 0–1, and that was that. Three lost World Cup finals, after the ones in 1974 and 1978.

I was having a chat afterwards, when I heard a noise outside.

'Fernando, Fernando, they're fighting!'

I said I was too busy. Besides, I'd been in too many fights before. Not this time, please. I was also feeling a bit down, because we'd just missed a unique opportunity to become the best footballing country in the world. Yes, it affected me! I'm Dutch and still a lover of football . . .

'Fernando! You *have* to come outside, it's really kicking off!'

As I walked out – duty called – I could see one poor bastard being beaten to a pulp by about 100 men. He had been provoking the crowd by waving a Spanish flag, so this was what they thought he deserved. It was mayhem.

Later on, I found out there had been more behind it. It had been the culmination of a feud between some trailer trash from the industrial town of Beverwijk and a group of Turkish and Moroccan youths. The guy with the flag was now ambushed; he couldn't go anywhere. He was about to be butchered.

I knew the boy. I was shocked. He was one of the freefighters I'd met at the gym. But one freefighter can't beat the shit out of a group that size. His little brother, who tried to help him, got severely battered too. Nobody came out to help him. So it was up to me. I went in and pushed a few of the assailants away. And I didn't just push: good old Fighting Spirit was using his fists too! I managed to grab the poor victim and drag him into my bar. He was barely alive.

Much later people asked me why I'd done it and hadn't I been afraid. The answer was no, I wasn't afraid. I didn't have the time to be afraid. It was instinct, pure instinct. A hero? Me? Well, without my intervention, the kid would be dead. So, you decide.

I'd been in a lot of fights, but this one was the worst. A hundred against one! That's worse than just unfair. No excuse for it. If I see something like that the streetfighter in me jumps out. I can't stand injustice. That's the reason why I smashed Radimov's face at Zenit, remember?

One of the reasons why I wasn't working at Se7en every day was the fact that I'd started to miss football. I'd called my brother Pedro. Maybe he could do something about it. And he could. On Tuesdays and Thursdays I was invited to train with EHC, my very first club, where, in the meantime, Pedro had become coach of the reserves. Back at EHC after thirty years!

It was a two-and-a-half-hour drive from Alkmaar – a five-hour round trip – but I still did it. I loved it. It was great to be on the grass again, albeit in Hoensbroek and not in Glasgow with 60,000 nutters around me! And I hadn't lost any of my skills. After a few months I even felt like a footballer again!

The big difference this time was that I was very careful not to hurt anybody. After all, they were amateurs, hobbyists with a full-time job. And I was their guest.

As an extra bonus, the bond with my brother Pedro, at whose place I crashed out, was getting stronger. I realised how much I'd missed him! Thanks to me being the world's biggest egomaniac, we had become completely alienated from each other. And Graciela didn't like my family at all, so she couldn't act like some kind of cement either.

The change had come on Thursday, 3 April 2008, quarter-finals of the UEFA Cup. We thrashed Bayer Leverkusen 1–4. Unfortunately I wasn't playing that night, but it was a memorable evening for me.

Pissed off that he couldn't get in touch with me, Pedro drove from Heerlen to Leverkusen. Not so much to watch the game, but to see his estranged brother – the brother he missed so much. I didn't know he would be there that night. Once again I had a new phone number, and once again I hadn't given it to him.

Normally punters can't get close to the players before and after a European match. The UEFA officials wanted us to get into the bus without any hassle, so we were totally shielded from the crowd. Well, that works for your average spectator, but not for Pedro. I was about to enter the coach, and there he was. My kid brother.

My little sibling, who had just climbed over a fence.

Nobody stopped him; it was as if it had to be this way. I immediately hugged him and gave him my shirt, the one that was free of sweat. I was so happy to see him after all those years . . . There and then I said to myself that I would never ever let him go again. Reunited – and it felt so good!

I gave him my number, and I got his. It was the start of something beautiful. No, the continuation of something beautiful! We kept our mutual promise. He often visited me in Saint Petersburg. I arranged a couple of tickets for him for the UEFA Cup Final in Manchester. We were inseparable again.

I cherish those moments, especially the memory of our trip to New York together, in 2001. I'd planned to go with Graciela, but she dropped out at the last moment. We'd probably had one of our many fights, I can't remember. Anyway, I didn't want this to ruin my trip, so I changed her ticket and booked one for Pedro. He absolutely loved it. I think it was his first business-class flight. To make the trip even more memorable for him, I booked us a couple of rooms in the Waldorf Astoria. You know, the one where Eddie Murphy shot Coming to America. Amazing location, close to Fifth Avenue and Central Park.

It was three days of total madness. We got pissed together every single night. Stayed in our expensive beds all day in an attempt to sober up, then drank so much we were literally bouncing off those beautiful stairs. As I was a wealthy footballer at the time, we could stuff ourselves with the most expensive champagne. We were Seriously Big Spenders. I even hired a limousine, in which we were driven through the city. The friggin' thing was about twenty feet long!

At four in the morning we were chewing on chicken wings, somewhere in a dark cave in the heart of the Bronx. We felt unassailable. How had we ended up there? We just jumped into a car and told the couple inside that they had to take us to 'a restaurant'. Madness, I know! So they took us to NY's most dangerous hood . . .

'Don't panic, guys,' the couple told us. 'We're sure you won't get shot.'

Totally irresponsible.

Now, I'm a sucker for a good piece of chicken, but preferably not under those circumstances. Pedro was shitting himself too. He wanted to get straight back to the hotel. But I had the munchies. And wasn't food why we were here in the first place? Let's give it a try, I suggested. And into the chicken joint we went, only to find out that . . . we were the only white people there! It was like being in a crazy movie! Yup, Pedro, never a dull moment with you! And boy, those chicken legs were delicious!

At one point, it looked as if Pedro was going to play in Glasgow too. Not at Rangers, but at Partick Thistle. They thought he would make a fine right-wing defender. All he had to do was sign.

No disrespect to Partick Thistle, but I advised him not to do it. Because I knew he would get homesick. Just like when he was living in Alkmaar for a while, when he was playing for the AZ reserves. 'You can't just drive from Glasgow to Heerlen,' I told him. Obvious, I know. But he wouldn't get rich at Partick Thistle either. 'Two thousand euros a month, at most. And you just had a little baby, bro!'

So he didn't sign. Our Pedro is a family man. Much more than I am. He would have suffered a lot in Glasgow. I'm much more of a loner than he is. Besides, he hadn't made it at AZ and Fortuna, so how was the kid going to survive in a match against Glasgow Rangers?

During my second stint with EHC, I kept driving down and up to Limburg. The times Pedro and I couldn't stand each other had long gone. We were so close now, we were like, er, brothers. I even became the godfather of his baby boy Dean, whom I had hardly seen during my years abroad. I loved going to the little chap's birthday and I saw that Pedro loved it too. My brother had become my comrade.

And, because of this new situation, I also got my mother and stepfather back. The two of them had never liked Graciela, so in previous years there hadn't been any contact. I had chosen my wife – as you do. Now, I was delighted that Mum liked Veronika.

Yes, it felt good to be back home, after all those years. I should've reached out for my family a lot earlier. But I was too scared. Too scared to be rejected.

The first occasion on which I saw them all again wasn't a happy one though. It was at my grandfather's funeral, my mother's old man. Pedro called me and asked me to come. Then, there was still a bit of friction, but I decided to do it anyway. I owed this to him. He had always been a great companion to me, an inspiration.

I found it a lot more significant than the cremation of my own father, Hein, four years earlier. Pedro went to the funeral, even though it was his birthday. I didn't care. Didn't know the bloke. Didn't even know where he lived. Huub, my stepfather, had always been my real dad. Huub had always been there for me. My biological father? I think I've seen him twice in my life. And I wasn't the only one who skipped his last farewell. Ten people showed up after the death of the old alcoholic.

I was so glad my mother accepted me again, in 2011. Also because we'd just found out that Veronika was pregnant. The thought that I had to tell my little daughter that she couldn't see her own granny was unbearable. We still have to talk things through, Mum and me, but at least we've made a start.

I know she hasn't been proud of me all her life and I know I have caused her a lot of sadness and pain, while she did everything she could to give me a good childhood. Yes, when I think about that, I feel ashamed.

Apart from my trips to Hoensbroek, I drove to Zeist as well. That's where the HQ of the Dutch FA is. I was studying there to become a football manager myself, because, yes, I really did miss the sport after all. I loved the idea of educating and teaching young kids, see if I could turn them into professionals-to-be. That was going to be my new challenge.

So there I was, back in the wonderful world of professional football! And what a nasty world it is. I noticed it immediately. Behind my back, people were saying to each other that Fernando Ricksen was the last person on earth who should become a football manager. He isn't qualified at all, they whispered. The fighter, the alcoholic, the nutcase – what kind of an example is he for those kids!

I ignored them. The course was tough though. I've worked with world-class coaches such as Willem van Hanegem, Dick Advocaat and Louis van Gaal, so I know a thing or two about football, but the theoretical part of the course was bothering me. There was so much reading to do. And that's not an easy thing for somebody who left school at sixteen and never did his homework. I found it hard to concentrate. I'd put the books aside every five minutes. But I didn't give up. I showed willpower. I tried and tried. Finally, thanks to my Fighting Spirit, I succeeded and received my diploma.

For my scholarship I went to the Fortuna youth team. I didn't feel like going to AZ and being confronted by all those bastards who still hated me. I didn't have those problems at Fortuna. They loved me there. That's one of the reasons that I look upon Fortuna Sittard as the most beautiful football club in the world.

Our matches were at 8 a.m. on Saturday mornings. I didn't mind. It felt like a warm bath.

There was only one thing that I didn't understand. Fortuna's main team were doing really badly in the Jupiler League, Holland's Second Division (the former First Division, to make it easier for you). According to the table, they were the worst professional football club in the land. I didn't agree. I saw the guys train at times and they really weren't that much worse than RKC Waalwijk, who were number one in the league.

It gave me heartache to see Fortuna suffer so much. They deserved better. The players did, and so did the fans. After the umpteenth defeat, I said to myself: I have to help this club!

In the meantime, back at Se7en strange things were happening too. Brilliant nights were followed by total disasters. Or so I was told. But it wasn't true. I was being robbed – by my own employees. The nights I wasn't there were just as busy as always; it was just that they told me they weren't. And when I checked the accounts I knew it for sure: they had been taking me for a ride! So I fired the bastards.

That felt good, but my problems weren't over yet. Thanks to their theft, I got into difficulties with the taxation department. Unpaid bills were piling up, and I was confronted with one debt collection agency after the other. This wasn't fun any more. This wasn't the life of a pub owner I had dreamt about. It was a complete disaster. Here was the proof that I wasn't qualified for the job at all. Inexperienced Fernando had made a mess out of things once again. And he needed help.

The only man I could think about at this stage was Tjerk Vermanen – a freefighter, yup, I knew a few! He had a lot of experience in running bars and stuff. But as much as he tried to help me, it was too late. The damage had been done already. And in the autumn of 2011, Se7en went bankrupt. The dream was over. And 300,000 euros had gone down the drain. What a waste.

Luckily I still had the two loves of my life: Veronika and football.

EIGHTEEN

RETURN

THE AWKWARD SITUATION FORTUNA Sittard was in kept worrying me. I could hardly sleep, to tell you the truth. If nobody did anything about it, the club could be finished within months. The demise of two-time Cup winner Fortuna – they grasped the thing in 1957 and 1964 – would be a disaster. For me, for Limburg, for Dutch football. How could it be stopped?

I couldn't stop fretting. Then, one morning in October, I got it! While I didn't have enough cash left to give Fortuna a financial injection, there was one thing I could give them. No, two things. My feet.

After a retirement of fifteen months and at the tender age of 34, I decided to make my comeback as a professional footballer. Well, it was better than just watching the ship sink.

Not that they hadn't asked me before. In August 2010 technical manager Fred van Barneveld had talked about it in a one-to-one with me. I'd decided not to do it. I was too heavy at the time, wasn't in shape. And, more to the point, I was enjoying my life without the ball. I was going on all these foreign trips with Veronika, and thanks to them I felt better than ever.

Another thing that stopped me was the thought of failure. I didn't want to be another big star who returns to his old club just to fall flat on his face. I didn't want to be another casualty.

Three months later, things were completely different. I now felt the need to do something. Especially after a flirtation with a Qatari sheikh and a hazy Brazilian investment company went absolutely nowhere. The dude in the white robe backed out at the last moment.

So, one morning in November I called Fortuna's head coach Wim Dusseldorp. Earlier on, he'd expressed his doubts about a possible comeback, but this time I gave him, well, the benefit of the doubt.

'Wim, I want to watch the first team's training sessions.'

Dusseldorp was full of enthusiasm. 'Bring your boots with you, Fernando, so you can join in!'

That was a bit premature. Still, I put the shoes in my bag, just in case . . .

I stepped in, and it went quite well. Dusseldorp was happy too, and told me I could be an addition to the team. I saw that he meant it. We agreed that I had to be careful. You never know how a body will react.

One potential problem wasn't a problem: the Russian FA told me I was free to do whatever I wanted to do. Money wasn't a problem either. Okay, I wasn't going to have a Russian or Scottish salary, but we came to an agreement, just like that. And I did the talking on my own, without Rob Jansen. This time I wasn't going after the jackpot.

Nothing could stop me now!

Come December, and I had a contract until the end of the season, with an option for another year. In return for my kicks and dribbles, I would receive 2,000 euros net. That was just petrol money – and for the rental of my house in Maaseik, Belgium – but, once again, it excluded any bonuses for games we won! Fifty euros per victory.

But I wasn't in it for the money. I was here to help Fortuna. And I was happy to be able to play football again. It was nice to earn what I earned with Rangers and Zenit, but I've never been a victim of materialism. That's because of my background. We didn't have expensive furniture or electronics. We had a fridge, that was the most important thing! And inside the fridge there was stuff to eat and drink.

Despite what you might think, I've never sought luxury. I was an exception, especially in Russia. While I preferred a bottle of good champagne, most of my colleagues just spent, spent, spent on the most expensive cars, houses, jewellery and gadgets. Seriously, that's what happens when you earn six million euros a year . . . Even so, some of my teammates would complain that another player was getting more than them. 'Coach, I think it's unfair that Anatoliy Tymoshchuk earns six million a year and I get a few million less!' It was pathetic.

I found it amusing to see how they squandered their cash. When we were in Noordwijk with Zenit, at a training camp, I sometimes took a taxi with Andrey Arshavin, Igor Denisov and Aleksandr Anyukov in order to go to P.C. Hooftstraat, the Fifth Avenue of Amsterdam. On our way back, they had so much stuff we'd need a second cab!

It was all Armani, Louis Vuitton, Gucci, Prada, Versace. And the logo had to be visible. Then they could show off back home.

The guys absolutely loved P.C. Hooftstraat. It was the main attraction of Amsterdam to them. While the city has so much else to offer! Like the Banana Bar, for instance, where you can eat fruit out of a girl's . . . Okay, enough of that!

I wanted to take them there, but soon changed my mind after a remark Arshavin once made. He said, 'I know why you love being with us, in Russia.'

'Oh, why?' I asked.

He pointed at a crowd of Dutch women who were passing by. Every single one of them was ugly. With all due respect, the way Dutch women dress is not attractive. Hair in a ponytail, feet in a pair of Uggs and off we go. The complete opposite to the stylish Russians.

So, okay, better not take them to a Dutch porn show. It would only disappoint. I mean, when you're used to the beauty of the Côte d'Azur, why would you swim in the North Sea?

Instead, I took them to the notorious Cooldown Café in the centre of Amsterdam, a party pub that I remembered from my AZ days. They were having the time of their lives. Not because of the women, but because of the booze – lots of it.

They were downing little shots at a ridiculous speed. Now, Arshavin is a bit of a garden gnome, size-wise, so at a certain moment I lifted him up and sat him on top of the bar. From there, the guy threw his empty glasses into the crowd, like a bowler at a cricket game. It was a miracle nobody got hurt.

The reason why he had enjoyed himself so much, he told me afterwards, was that nobody recognised him. Nobody had asked him for an autograph or a photo. He could be completely himself.

Still, a night like that was an exception. Most of the time when abroad, the Russians were only interested in shopping. I didn't – and still don't – care about price tags. I never buy terribly expensive stuff. Okay, I admit it: I had a 10,000-euro Rolex and a 200,000-euro Ferrari, but the car was second-hand.

Food and drink, that's where most of my money went.

Did I finally end up in Belgium as a tax exile? Not at all. It was because of Veronika. Because she's Russian, she couldn't just move to Holland. First, they wanted her to go back to Saint Petersburg to do a Dutch 'acclimatisation course'. Bullshit, but those are the rules. All in all, it would cost us three months. We didn't fancy the idea. So when we heard it was a lot easier south of the border, we took off. In Belgium you had to do a similar course, but at least you could do it there. You didn't have to go back to Russia.

That's why we moved to Maaseik. And because it's very close to Sittard. The region is even called 'Belgian Limburg'. We had a lovely house there, with a big garden, and it was only a fifteen-minute drive from Fortuna. Ideal.

And to top things off, Veronika passed her exams just like that and received her residence permit. Still, she was struggling. Of course she was. Life in Belgium is different from that in Russia. Some people think that moving from Western Europe to Eastern Europe is going from good to bad. In the case of Saint Petersburg it's the other way around! Saint Petersburg is a rich and modern metropolitan city. To swap that for Maaseik with its 25,000 sleepy inhabitants is not easy.

We missed the 24-hour lifestyle of Saint Petersburg. I mean, sometimes we went out for dinner in the middle of the night there. Try to get a steak in Maaseik after nine? Impossible. All the shops close at six. And on Sundays they don't even open!

So, I began having my usual doubts again. Was it too soon? Should I have let her stay in Saint Petersburg a little bit longer? And why were we in Maaseik?

No, my sweetheart said to me, it was going to be all right. She just needed a bit more time to get used to things. I shouldn't worry so much. Still, I gave her regular flight tickets so that she could see her mother as much as possible.

I soon sensed that those brief trips to Russia had a positive effect on Veronika. Every time she came back, she was shining like the sun above my Spanish villa. And after a while she even grew to enjoy life in Maaseik. She made her own friends and so on. It was brilliant to see. Fewer trips to Saint Petersburg were needed, and we began doing more and more things together. We'd jump in the car and drive all the way to Brussels, for instance. And when we finally had the internet, she could Skype her mum.

Now that I was playing on a professional basis again, I had to abandon my manager's course. They demanded that I train various amateur teams all over the country, but I simply couldn't combine that with my job at Fortuna. I tried it, but I couldn't stand the fact that it meant coming home late every bloody time. I didn't want to do that to Veronika.

Fortuna had to play away games in Veendam and Emmen, up north in the Netherlands. Veendam was the furthest away of them all. They've now gone, but their stadium was called De Langeleegte, meaning 'the long emptiness'. A very appropriate name!

We spent hours on the bus, as Fortuna didn't own a private plane, but I loved being on the road. It was pointless comparing Fortuna with Zenit. And why would I? Why should I think about world-class players like Arshavin, Danny, Denisov, Malafeev, Dominguez or Fayzulin when I was going towards stadium De Baandert with my boots and shin pads? I would just make myself tense.

So, on my way to the Meerdijk ground of FC Emmen, I wasn't thinking about the times that I checked in at the Kempinsky or the Ritz-Carlton prior to a clash with a bunch of Moscow millionaires. I was now a member of Fortuna Sittard, the worst team in Holland's Second Division. Fortuna players don't stay in hotels; they drive home in the hours after the game. Simple as that. Football at its purest. Loved it!

Some minor irritations were creeping in, however. For instance, I couldn't stand the mentality of some of our younger players. Checking your iPhone instead of joining a group talk? Well, that's disrespectful and not very professional, in my opinion, but carry on. But, please carry some balls and cones to the training field like everybody else. You're not feeling above that, I hope, as a simple Fortuna player!

Yes, they did. They didn't even look at the cones and vests that lay there, ready to be taken to the training pitch. Different generation. But I told them what I thought about their behaviour, and judging by the way they stared at me, they didn't like what I said.

They were pussies, most of them. Didn't have any of my Fighting Spirit. A total lack of the good old over-my-dead-body mentality. A lack of skills too. Some of them couldn't even kick a ball straight. And they weren't even drunk, like Arshavin!

Some of them really weren't qualified for professional football. And that's what I told them in a group meeting. They didn't appreciate that, especially kids like Wouter Scheelen and Kévin Diaz. They thought I just wanted to take the piss out of them, because I didn't like them.

I did give them the odd, let's call it 'push', and, yes, I did shout at them, more than I did with the others, but that was because I wanted them to get better. Because I believed in them. I wasn't teasing you, boys!

Nevertheless, they had different ideas, and at one point they did a Radimov behind my back and complained about me. Ridiculous, totally ridiculous, and it didn't get them anywhere. Let's face it. Have you heard of Wouter Scheelen and Kévin Diaz? There you go!

Things were different now. Fifteen years earlier, players used to laugh at times. Now they were all engrossed with their smartphones, the moment they were off the pitch. Football humour had died out completely.

This was a task for Fernando!

In order to put the fun back into Fortuna, I made a plan. And not a vulgar one. I didn't want to be like Paul Gascoigne, who used to fill up the bath with a ridiculous amount of bubble bath, not because he liked to be super-clean but to hide the fact that he'd had a crap in the water. After having a shit, he'd jump out, leaving the floating turd for the next guy, mostly a youngster, and say, 'Enjoy the bubble bath, mate, I put a little bit extra in it!'

I didn't find that amusing at all. Or pissing against your legs in the shower when your eyes are closed, which they do in Holland. I never found that funny either.

What I did was cut out some newspaper headlines which I stuck onto the players' lockers. There was a suitable headline for everyone.

Ricky Geenen, a young defender with a sense of humour and self-awareness, found the header 'I AM UGLY, BUT NEVERTHELESS HAPPY'. He got it!

One of the best ones was for Joeri Schroyen. He once had to skip training because he had to help his uncle pick up some old iron. I remembered something about a theft at the local chemical company DSM: 'TWENTY THOUSAND TONS OF IRON STOLEN'.

I was in stitches, and finally people were laughing again. And, more important, the guys picked it up. One day I found a clipping on my own locker that said: 'MONEY DOESN'T MAKE YOU HAPPY'.

Mission accomplished!

I always made sure nobody suffered from my pranks. Only once did I fail, with our caretaker Marco Lemmens. He very nearly had a heart attack, and it was all my fault.

Because I didn't only give but also received – we're talking about hard kicks on the legs here, reader – I played every match with an injection of Diclofenac, an anti-inflammatory. Without it, I would've

225

been out of my rhythm after every single whack. Diclofenac made me feel great, for at least three hours. It was always the same ritual: I dropped my pants, the doc put an imaginary cross on my bum and in went the needle. Simple as that. Anyone could do that.

Well, not quite . . .

Because of the fact that Fortuna isn't a super-rich professional club with its own medical staff, our Kick Hamers sometimes had to be at his workplace, in the hospital. That left me two choices: forget about the injection or choose somebody else to violate my buttocks.

Marco Lemmens wanted to give it a try. Anyway, I thought, this is a perfect moment for a good joke! So I dropped my pants, like I always did, and told him about the imaginary cross. 'About there.'

He nodded.

'But not too hard, otherwise things could go seriously wrong.'

Up till then, things had been going well. In the fourteen games when I'd been part of the team, we had beaten the likes of Sparta, FC Emmen and RBC. So Marco did exactly what the patient ordered. Right spot, not too hard, not too soft either . . . not too deep. He looked relieved.

Until I started to scream. 'Ow! Ow! Ow! Ow! Ow! Ouch!' I looked at him as if I could kill him. 'Marco, what the hell have you done? I can't feel anything any more! You've paralysed me! I'll never play football again!'

His face turned as white as Bing Crosby's Christmas. He really thought he'd screwed it up.

'Joke!' I laughed.

No, not that funny actually, if you look back at it.

Another over-the-top incident was the time we put tiger balm into Marc Wagemaker's socks. Normally we did this with underpants, but after a while everybody became too suspicious, so we decided to go for another item of clothing. Unfortunately we put too much of the stuff in his socks and he burned both his feet. He was out of the team for a while.

The rest of Fortuna were hot too. We played better and won more games than before my arrival. On that memorable day, 13

December 2011, we immediately beat RKC Waalwijk (3–2). No surprise to me, as I knew we had the quality! It was the first away victory since, er, the previous one, which had been 31 matches ago.

Despite being nervous, I played a good game. Maybe I was still a little overweight, but I didn't have any difficulties with my direct opponent, Donny de Groot. And at the end of the season, we were in sixteenth place. Okay, not enough for a triumphant ticker-tape parade, but at least we weren't the ugly ducklings of Dutch football any more.

A year later, we were in eleventh place, followed by a ninth place in the 2012/13 season. We even made it to the play-offs then! It had been quite a climb from the cellar! More to the point, Fortuna had been saved from tumbling down to the amateur section. Had that happened the club would have been bankrupt.

I felt proud that I had helped to stop that process. The fans were grateful too. They realised I was not some kind of pensionado who had just come down to earn a few bob. One particular supporter even made a calculation. The outcome was that Fortuna had gained most points when I was playing. It made me as proud as a peacock.

Yeah, Fortuna supporters are the best in the world. Wait a minute! Didn't I say that about Rangers fans earlier? What a lucky bastard to have played for both teams, then!

Anyway, the Fortuna crowd always managed to cheer me up. Like on 26 April 2013, just before the confrontation with FC Dordrecht. Due to a back injury I wasn't playing, so I was about to watch the match from the stands.

There was something in the air. I could feel it. A buzz. Something was going on where the Tifosi Giallo Verde were gathered. Those were the guys who always called me Fernando le Commando. There was a bit of green and yellow moving, but I couldn't work it out.

Suddenly I saw ropes. They hadn't been there before. Well, okay, never mind. The match was about to begin and I took a gulp of coffee. I almost choked. Not because the coffee was too hot. No, it was the noise that freaked me out. All of a sudden they'd started to make this enormous racket. And up it went, this *huge* banner! It was at least thirty feet wide and thirty feet high. On it were my face and my name.

It was like looking in a giant mirror. Because, in all honesty, they'd done a great job! It was really me they had painted, not Captain Birdseye.

I was so emotional I even forgot to applaud. So I do it for you now, wonderful fans of Fortuna Sittard!

Anyway, to all those people who kept asking me whether I didn't find it sad that I was playing there, instead of in big stadiums in Scotland and Russia: no, no regrets at all! I loved football and I loved Fortuna, so I was at the right place.

Just too bad that I . . . Yes, you've guessed it, another conflict with a manager loomed! This time it was Tiny Ruijs, the successor of Wim Dusseldorp. One of the nicest and friendliest people in Dutch football, I had always liked him, ever since I was in Fortuna's youth teams. That's why I decided to warn him about his two assistants, Fuat Usta and Roel Coumans. I suspected them of preparing a coup.

Tiny didn't believe me when I told him. Well, at least I'd warned him. That was all I could do.

Last game of the season, Eindhoven away (that's EVV Eindhoven, not its bigger cousin PSV), and Suat Usta, brother of Fuat, was standing next to me. A bigger dribbler than a newborn baby. I passed the ball to him. He started running, lost it, Eindhoven scored. They eventually won the match 4–3.

The indifference of the guy got on my nerves. I started yelling at him during the break. To my surprise Tiny supported him. 'Don't curse, Fernando.'

'What? *Wait* a minute . . . So it was *my* fault? What's happening here? Are you trying to say that I . . . It was Suat's fault, not mine! That's exactly what you have to tell him. And if you don't have the guts to do that, I'll do it for you!'

'Fernando, you're out.'

'Sooo . . . are we the big bad manager all of a sudden? What a brave man! Tell me, who exactly is the boss in this dressing room: you or those two sidekicks of yours?'

Silence.

Fifteen minutes later everybody had gone. And I was still there, totally on my own. Me, who had wanted to protect his manager.

A week later, against Go Ahead Eagles, I started on the bench. What a humiliation.

Still, we talked it out, Fortuna and me, and that's why I started my third season with them. Which lasted no more than eight games. After that, my back was killing me. I shouldn't have started that third season at all.

I think it was because of Fortuna's dodgy pitches, which were as hard as concrete. They left me with a hernia, and I had to get surgery for it. After the operation, in February, I tried to fight back, but I didn't succeed.

At that point, I was just happy that I could walk! Now that was something that had *really* worried me. I remember one terrible morning, in December . . . the morning after the slide before. I had fallen on the hard surface and now, in bed, I couldn't move my leg at all.

I was freaking out.

Veronika looked at me with her big, questioning eyes. It was true: my right leg was completely paralysed! And no, it wasn't just asleep, as happens to everybody once in a while. In that case you can still move the bloody thing. Now I couldn't.

The next image I had was that of me in a wheelchair. Career over. Couldn't even become a manager any more.

I called the doctor, who told me it could be a hernia. Six weeks of rest and I would be all right again. And, yes, after a while I could walk again. But it dawned on me that my footballing days were over. No, they *had* to be over. It was enough. No more risks, no more pain. One day in March I decided: thank you very much, that's it.

Looking back, my last ever match was the one on 16 November 2012. It was a home defeat against Sparta, 1–3. After an hour I was replaced by the Belgian, Ramazan Çevik. And that was it.

I didn't cry, the day I took the decision to stop playing football.

'Why should I?' I said to Veronika. 'I'm not dying!'

My life wasn't over yet. This day, as they say, was the beginning of the rest of it; the beginning of something else, something new.

My retirement was big news. 'FORMER INTERNATIONAL RICKSEN CALLS IT A DAY' was the headline on Teletext. Despite my terrible behaviour in the past, I was still somebody. Holland still respected me.

Meanwhile I'd become a completely different person. I realised there was life after football. It was a life with my dear one, Veronika. We spent a lot of time together in Maaseik. No more drunken antics. I had completely calmed down. Calmed down and settled down.

We even spoke about having a baby. And it wasn't all talk and no action, because on 6 June 2012 our beautiful little daughter Isabella Kristina was delivered. She was born right after my youth team had won a tournament. While having a victory dinner in a Chinese restaurant, Veronika's belly started to rumble. So we said goodbye to the crowd and raced to the hospital.

The moment I had Isabella in my arms, I immediately realised she was a special child. Okay, all parents say that about their own offspring, but this was really the case. Just think about it: a Dutch baby, born in Belgium to a Russian mother. It could be less complicated!

Actually it is more complicated. Isabella has a half-brother named Lars. Born on 11 December 1999, in Alkmaar. I was playing for AZ then, and never had any contact with the boy.

I'd only had sex with his mother twice; it was lust, not love. Maaike slipped a piece of paper with her phone number on it under my windshield wiper. I hesitated for quite some time, but eventually I decided to call her. We got together twice: once with a condom, once without.

A few months later I saw her again. This time she wasn't alone. She was pregnant.

'Is it mine?' I asked.

'Yes.'

I was angry with her. She'd known this for weeks already and only now did she decide to share the news with me. I told her I didn't want to be with her and put a large sum of money in a bank account. It was the most I could do.

C'mon, how could I have raised a child while I was a professional footballer? I was 22 and never at home. I was much too young to be a responsible father and I didn't have a stable relationship.

During his childhood I didn't want to bother Lars. When he is an adult, I would love to meet him and explain to him why I didn't see him for all those years. I hope he'll understand, but I know it won't be easy.

NINETEEN

RESIGNATION

'SO, LOOKING BACK, DON'T you regret the fact that, thanks to your wildness and stupidity, your career hasn't been as successful as it could have been?'

That's what people keep asking me. It's a difficult question to answer. What if I had been, let's say, a Mark van Bommel? Dunno. Maybe. I've played twelve games for the national team. Could've been more. Could've been less.

My problem has always been that I needed an outlet. Otherwise I would start to think and think and, eventually, tense up. Completely. I needed to let steam off – a lot. Without that outlet I wouldn't have been of any use to a manager

Family man Mark lived purely for his sport. I needed distraction to play at the highest level. But I agree, I've overdone it a bit, with the booze, the drugs, the girls. It was my way of dealing with the situation. After a night of partying, my head would be empty again. Otherwise I would have thought about the previous match non-stop and it would've driven me insane.

Yes, I burned a Mount Everest of money, but at least I had a good time doing it.

Still, there is one thing that I wish I hadn't done. I shouldn't have done coke during my last months in Russia. That scarred me for life. Look at my CV and you'll notice there's a year missing: the

2009/10 season – the season in which I didn't play a single match. I've always said that I lost interest in football in that period, that I wasn't motivated because I didn't like the game any more, but that was a lie. I was suspended, after snorting cocaine, two weeks before the Europa League play-off match against Nacional Madeira, on 20 August 2009.

I wasn't even anxious when they checked me that night on the Portuguese flower island. The toot had been two weeks ago, so fat chance they'd find any traces of it in my urine. I even grinned as I pissed. I wasn't thinking about a possible worst-case scenario. No, I was happy. Happy that I was finally back with the squad again, on a European trip. Never expected that from Dick's successor Davydov. After all, my last European match had been nine months ago, an away game against BATE Borisov. Against Real Madrid and Juventus I had been *persona non grata*.

I looked upon my presence in Madeira as a small ray of sunshine in the Cold War between Davydov and me, as the possible beginning of something new. Why else did he take me with him?

That was then. Three days later we had our argument at the bottom of the stairs in the hotel. Followed by *that* phone call from our doctor.

After a few fruitless attempts he finally caught me on the phone. He didn't waste any time: 'You've tested positive.' UEFA had found traces of cocaine in my urine and that was the end of the line for me. I was suspended for a full year.

I was completely blown away. Not being allowed to play football was more difficult than my battle with the bottle. Football was my life. From the tender age of four, all I did was kick a ball. As a kid I always came home after dark, due to an agreement with my parents. As long as the streetlights were off, I was allowed to stay out. I was that passionate about football. And all those years later it was taken away from me. I was devastated.

Yes, it was my own fault. I shouldn't have taken the damn stuff. Apart from being an athlete, I was a role model for kids, so it was a very bad thing to do. I want to say to everybody who is reading this: *don't do coke!* Don't do hard drugs. They're poison and they'll ruin you, even if you don't notice it. They'll destroy your life, your career, everything.

Nonetheless I didn't agree with the penalty. I mean, I hadn't taken the drug to perform better on the pitch. It was recreational. I wasn't a cyclist in the Tour de France, preparing to climb Mont Ventoux. I was an off-duty football player with personal problems. A little bit of understanding, please!

The suspension made me suicidal. Not that I've ever climbed to the top of a bridge, ready to jump, but it was close. To distract myself I opened that pub in Alkmaar, but we all know how that ended.

The fact that I'm still here is purely thanks to Veronika. She dragged me out of my misery – and I am so grateful for that. She really is my guardian angel. She supported me day and night, when running away would've been the easiest option. Once again, Veronika, thank you very, very much! I love you.

And I can assure you it was tough for her too! I had become completely lethargic. I'd lie on the sofa watching a movie without really noticing I was watching a movie, if you catch my drift. My mind was miles away.

'Nobody knows you when you're down and out', is the title of an old blues song. Not true, not in my case. People kept calling me, dropping by to ask if I needed anything. But I couldn't accept their help. I didn't want to bother them. It was my misery and I had to deal with it myself. That's what I thought. I didn't realise that due to that attitude I was starting to lose them.

Only much later, when I was working with the Fortuna youth team, did the sun start to shine again. And in order to keep the dark clouds away once and for all, I asked for professional help, just as I had done four years earlier when I visited the Sporting Chance Clinic.

I joined Alcoholics Anonymous, in Amsterdam, and this time I didn't have any doubts. I was just a bit scared that I wouldn't be 'Anonymous' for long, being the former football hero that I was.

But there was no need to worry. In the Lucas Church in Osdorp, life didn't rotate around Fernando Ricksen. Every single person was there for himself. Why should they care about other people's problems?

So once again I had to talk about my demons, all three of them this time: drink, drugs and depression. The meetings were soothing and made me drink a lot less. At a certain point, I no longer had alcohol in the house. I was on my way back. I was ready to enjoy life again.

Still, the battle rages on. You can't just be an ex-alcoholic overnight. You have to keep fighting the temptation. It's a short-time strategy. You can only say to yourself: I'm not having a drink today. You can't plan the rest of the week, let alone the rest of the year! That's useless.

Drugs I don't take at all any more. That is the only good thing that came out of the suspension. Women? Been there, done that, lost the T-shirt. I have Veronika and that is enough. My womanising days are over; for that reason you won't see me in bars or clubs. It was fun, but it's all in the past now. Besides, gold-diggers aren't interested in me now that I'm on normal wages!

Drink-wise, I still enjoy the occasional glass of wine at dinner. Well, nobody's perfect. But I am so strong nowadays that I can stop after one or two glasses. And I've never been plastered. I don't want to be. No, not quite true. Deep down inside I would love to drink myself silly, but at least I now know that I shouldn't. One day I hope to be totally clean. That is my next challenge. Being off booze completely would be as much a highlight as, for instance, the 2004/05 season, in which we won everything, with Rangers. The season that I ended up being best player in the league.

I feel privileged that I've played with some of the best footballers in the world. In the Dutch national team I had Van der Sar, Frank de Boer, Stam, Sneijder, Van der Vaart, Robben, Kluivert, Seedorf, Van Nistelrooy and Van Bommel around me. At AZ I played with Van Galen, Moens and Huiberts. My fellow Rangers were, among others, Caniggia, Flo, Amoruso, Ferguson, Ronald de Boer, Van

Bronckhorst and Moore. In Saint Petersburg there were Arshavin, Malafeev, Anyukov, Danny, Denisov and Tymoshchuk.

Not difficult to pick and choose an All Star Team from these names, is it?

And if you ask them about Fernando Ricksen, they will all say he's a nutcase, a total psycho, but he never let us down and always did his best to win the match. Some will even tell you I'm a sweet guy.

At RKSV Minor – what's in a name? – the modest amateur club where I started playing after my professional days were over, they've only seen the nice side of me. Okay, I still didn't want to lose, but I didn't kick anybody off the field any more. (Minor were trained by a certain Pedro Ricksen, for the record.)

Pedro had warned me: people are going to provoke you. Like they had been doing to him for years, being the brother of 'that alcoholic'. More than once Pedro gave in and whacked one of those creepy opponents, and received a red card as a result.

So, I had to ensure something like that wasn't going to happen during my stint with RKSV Minor. But it didn't mean I was going to tolerate a kick on my shin, oh no! You can have the pleasure of writing on Twitter or Facebook that you hurt Fernando Ricksen, but don't think I won't kick you back!

I've had my fair share of provocation, especially in Scotland. I broke my nose so often that I don't have a septum now. Try to squeeze it, it feels like a rubber duck! And I lost more teeth than you've seen in the movie *Jaws* – thanks to Craig Brewster, the battering ram of Dundee United. He once planted his elbow in my mouth, after which I spat out both of my front teeth. Continued to play, of course. Hey, it was my teeth, not my leg!

'Is it nice being Fernando Ricksen?' That's another thing people sometimes ask me. Depends on your perception of 'nice', is my standard answer. If you like an extreme life with very high highs and very low lows then yes, it was great fun to be me. But it was heavy at times, very heavy. That's why you can only handle it if you're blessed with the right spirit.

A Fighting Spirit.

Sure, I could blame a lot of people for the lows in my life. I could blame Graciela, for forbidding me to keep in touch with my family. I could blame various managers, for not letting me play. I could blame my friends, for giving me cocaine. But that wouldn't be fair. I am the only one to blame. I messed things up so much. It was me, and only me!

I am not proud of it. I know lots of you love to hear (and read, otherwise you wouldn't be on this page!) about my stupid past, but I sincerely regret parts of it. I have hurt people – loads of them. So, no, I'm not pleased with a lot of things that happened.

But at the same time, it has been a fruitful period with lots of trophies and titles. And look at me now! Look at what I've gathered, apart from all that silverware. I have a lovely wife, a beautiful daughter, a caring family, supportive friends and loyal supporters from Sittard to Glasgow.

So, back to what that psychologist at the Sporting Chance Clinic in Hampshire asked me: 'What is it exactly that you have achieved in your life?'

I now know the answer. All of the above, sir!

TWENTY

FIGHTING SPIRIT

ALL OF A SUDDEN, I realised something was wrong. It was my voice. It was different. I sounded like I was drunk. But I wasn't – absolutely not.

It was the summer of 2013 and I had reduced my alcohol intake to just two glasses of beer a week. Thanks to Veronika, Isabella and some treatment, I could keep myself under control. The difficulties with swallowing, the constant tiredness, the slurred speech; none of it had anything to do with my years of being an alcoholic. None of it. So what was it? Could it be something to do with the hernia? That's what I thought. No, that's what I *hoped*.

But soon my hopes were shattered. The moment I couldn't even ignite a simple cigarette lighter, I knew. This had nothing to do with a hernia. It was my muscles. There was something wrong with them.

That's what the doctors told me too. 'Something muscular.' But what exactly? They didn't know.

For a month I lived in uncertainty. Maybe it was going to be all right. Maybe it wasn't. It was one what-if after another.

I tried to push it from my mind and searched for some distraction, which I found, as always, with Veronika and Isabella, and with Fortuna Sittard, where I was still training young kids.

Then came October. The verdict. The one thing I didn't want

to hear. It was a death sentence. I had an incurable disease. A killer disease.

I had contracted motor neuron disease (MND), also known as ALS (amyotrophic lateral sclerosis). It is an illness which makes you lose control over one muscle after the other. Within a few years you kick the bucket, in normal cases.

Normal cases, yes. But I'm not a normal guy. I'm Fernando Ricksen.

I am a fighter, a warrior. Remember what they say at Rangers? No surrender! That goes for me too. I'm not going to give up, not just like that. Forget about it, Mr MND!

A motor neuron disease patient has a maximum of three years to live, that's what the doctors told me. My reply was, 'Don't count on it, guys,' because I simply refuse to go within those three years. I have too much left to live for.

Of course I'm scared at times. But I have good days as well. I take my medication and I sleep like a log.

The scientists don't know everything about the disease yet, and one day somebody will be the first person to beat it. Let me be that first person.

Me, Fernando Ricksen. The warrior also known as Fighting Spirit.

EPILOGUE

BY MICHAEL GRANT

SCOTTISH FOOTBALL CORRESPONDENT FOR *THE TIMES*

FERNANDO RICKSEN WAS true to his word. Fight MND? Boy did he fight it. At times the battle and effort to stay alive appeared almost superhuman. Long, long after the doctors and medical experts thought he would have surrendered to it Fernando was still there, still fighting. Initially he was given only 18 months to live and at that milestone he was still strong. Three years is another point that most sufferers do not reach. Fernando passed that too. And four years. And five.

Fernando lived his life in two acts with a crunching gear change which transformed everything. The diagnosis came just as his life was belatedly calming down and the joy and responsibility of parenthood were beginning. His precious Isabella was born in June, 2012, and the MND diagnosis came only 16 months later. The disease redefined Fernando. It completely altered how people saw and reacted to him. For those who already regarded him as a favourite, the affection dramatically deepened. For rival fans and others who had disliked or been neutral about him, the brutality of MND meant any negativity melted away.

As a player he was always a divisive figure – and didn't he revel in it – but his suffering united people in rapidly escalating warmth, respect and sympathy for what he was going through and how he was facing it all head-on. And that turnaround was instant. It was while Fernando was on television in Holland promoting the first edition of this book in 2013 that viewers, and the show's presenter, noticed he was slurring his words. His friend Vincent de Vries recalled the reaction on Twitter from those who were watching the programme – people were saying 'look at that arsehole, he's still drunk' – only for that to change in a matter of seconds as Fernando emotionally revealed why his speech had slowed. If the diagnosis changed his life, that television moment permanently changed everything about how people saw him.

It's a writer's cliché to call anyone with a terminal illness 'brave'. But what else to call a man who continued to put himself out there in the cause of raising funds and awareness so that he and others could take the fight to MND? Fernando began to devote himself to charity events in Holland and Scotland to generate funds. And every time he put himself in front of a crowd or the cameras he knew people were scrutinising him, however well-meaning they were, to see how the condition was weakening him.

It all got harder and harder. Of course, his condition deteriorated over time. Speaking and at times even breathing became difficult. His muscle function became ever more impaired. Gradually his mobility became more and more limited. He became wheelchair and eventually bed-bound. It was possible to fully communicate only via eye movements which were interpreted by a voice-computer. 'I just keep going, it's nothing special,' he said at one point. 'The people that take care of me do all the work. I just sit and tell them what to do.'

Gradually, naturally, inevitably, he looked a little thinner, weaker and more ill on each of his public appearances. It took enormous effort and courage to put himself out there at all but he would attend events and smile, pose for pictures, communicate and interact as best he could and drive auctions and raffles simply by being present, although he fed off the energy it created and cheekily confessed that he still loved the attention. Creating the Fernando Ricksen Foundation did more to raise awareness and funds. He lived with Veronika and Isabella at the family home near Valencia until becoming unwell at a fans' event in Glasgow in October, 2018, which led to a spell in hospital and acceptance that he was too ill to fly again. The charity events became too difficult for him to attend. His final nine months were spent in St Andrew's Hospice in Airdrie, a few miles outside Glasgow. Veronika and Isabella made as many trips to see him as they could. A picture of Isabella was always on the tray-table beside the computer screen.

Fernando died on 18 September, 2019. Survive for maybe 18 months? He fought for almost six years.

His clubs and his country had always done him proud. Fortuna Sittard staged a testimonial game for him in 2014, named a stand in his honour and erected a statue. In 2015, Rangers staged a benefit game which drew a crowd of over 42,000 and the door was open for him any time he wanted. The day after he died, Ibrox hosted a Europa League game against Feyenoord which doubled as a deeply poignant Fernando tribute night. An enormous shrine had grown consisting of scarves, shirts, flowers and flags for Fernando, spreading from Ibrox's iconic gates as fans arrived over the course of the days after his death to place something down and stand for a moment with their head bowed. Many of the mementos had loving, handwritten messages. Around 90 minutes before the Feyenoord game there was the astonishing sight of a guy walking through the mourning fans in a Celtic top, shorts and a baseball cap. Fernando would have loved the guy's sheer nerve. The Rangers fans parted slightly to let him through and after he placed a Celtic scarf among the tributes – one of many – they gave him a warm round of applause. He nodded his head solemnly then left.

That night, thousands turned up for the game not in Rangers blue but in the club's orange third kit, speckling Holland colours across the stands. There was a minute's silence for him before kick-off and a rousing applause in the second minute – he was their number two, after all – which brought the unprecedented spectacle of the players and coaches pausing to join in. A banner was raised in the Broomloan Road end: 'A warrior until the end, rest easy Fernando'. When Holland played Northern Ireland in Rotterdam a few days later both sets of fans chanted 'there's only one Fernando Ricksen' during a minute's applause. The crowds were also out to line the route of his funeral procession in Glasgow, which passed Ibrox. At the first Rangers home game after his funeral, against Aberdeen, fans raised over £23,000 and MND Scotland said it was the biggest total from a bucket collection in the charity's 38-year history.

Motor Neurone Disease is a neurodegenerative disorder. It is indiscriminate in terms of who it affects and inhumane in the endless cruelties it inflicts on sufferers. Some studies have suggested that intense physical activity can heighten the risk of developing MND and a number of prominent former footballers and other sports figures have been diagnosed. Fernando was blessed and lived life to the full and then had to endure a torture painfully witnessed by hundreds of thousands of supporters who were emotionally invested in his battle. For most of his life his large, handsome and expressive face showed fun, celebration and his sparkle and sense of mischief. Latterly it grew haunted and pained as he was entombed by MND. His sense of humour never left him but over time the tone changed in his infrequent charity appearances from 'fighting spirit' and being the man to 'beat' MND to simply attempting to have comfort and peace in his final days. The love of his family and closest friends meant he found that.

He couldn't beat MND but let's just say that by the end this grotesque disease knew it had been in a helluva game. As Fernando's world grew smaller the respect, sympathy and compassion for him spread to all who were even fleeting witnesses to his doomed struggle to stay alive. By the end he was never more loved.

CAREER TIMELINE

SEASON	CLUB	APPEARANCES	GOALS
1993/94	Fortuna Sittard	2	0
1994/95	Fortuna Sittard	30	2
1995/96	Fortuna Sittard	28	1
1996/97	Fortuna Sittard	34	4
1997/98	AZ Alkmaar	32	1
1998/99	AZ Alkmaar	31	0
1999/00	AZ Alkmaar	29	9
2000/01	Glasgow Rangers	27	1
2001/02	Glasgow Rangers	31	4
2002/03	Glasgow Rangers	35	3
2003/04	Glasgow Rangers	30	1
2004/05	Glasgow Rangers	38	4
2005/06	Glasgow Rangers	21	0
2006	Zenit St. Petersburg	14	2
2007	Zenit St. Petersburg	14	0
2008	Zenit St. Petersburg	8	0
2009	Zenit St. Petersburg	0	0
2010/11	Fortuna Sittard	17	0
2011/12	Fortuna Sittard	2	1
2012/13	Fortuna Sittard	8	0
Total		*452*	*33*

HONOURS

Netherlands	12 caps (0 goals)
Fortuna Sittard	First Division Champions 1995
AZ Alkmaar	First Division Champions 1998
Glasgow Rangers	SPL Champions 2003 and 2005
	Scottish Cup winners 2002 and 2003
	League Cup winners 2002, 2003 and 2005
Zenit St. Petersburg	Russian Champions 2007
	Russian Super Cup winners 2008
	UEFA Cup winners 2008
	European Super Cup winners 2008